PRAISE F

Every Storm Runs Out of Rain

"What's a leader to do to keep her team engaged in a crisis like a pandemic? Inspire. How should they do it? Be honest, be vulnerable, express gratitude, put things in perspective and communicate consistently.

As one of the recipients of Amy's weekly emails during the most difficult and uncertain times in the health care field, I can attest to the impact of the authentic and intentional weekly messages Amy shared with her team. The emails alone are a great model for any leader, but the content and reflections also provide an inside view into how one of the country's premier health care systems persevered during the pandemic."

— Cheryl Iverson, Corporate Director of Community Engagement, Emory Healthcare

"Amy's deep sense of responsibility and humanity were on full display during a once in a century pandemic. I had the privilege of reading her weekly letters in real time due to having a family member on her team. They are very thoughtfully written and incredibly inspiring and should serve as a valuable example of how to lead with heart and grace during difficult times. Amy is an immensely effective leader."

— Terri Goren, Principal, Goren & Associates LLC, Strategic Marketing and Communications Consulting

"The reflections are as powerful as the real-time messages and through the gift of hindsight, bring a new connection to today. What an incredible recounting of a remarkable time in our lives. *Every Storm Runs Out of Rain* provides authentic leadership lessons of encouragement, resilience, and a team-first focus at every turn. Learning straight from Amy's direct communications with those she led—all while navigating the global pandemic roller coaster at one of the world's leading academic health system, makes this book especially uplifting and poignant. As Amy shares in such an entertaining fashion, we must always remember this time in our lives and impact it had on us, our families, and our communities."

— Dane Peterson, Chief Operating Officer of Children's Health and Former President and CEO of Emory Healthcare

"*Every Storm Runs Out of Rain* is an absolute must-read for any leader needing a dose of inspiration. The lived experiences of Amy as she led her team and survived one of the darkest periods in our world history are captured poetically and realistically, uniquely drawing from phenomenal leaders past and present. It is compelling and brilliant in its ability to remind us that even in our most vulnerable times, we can find the strength to overcome life's biggest challenges."

— Sandra D. Mackey, Chief Marketing Officer, Bon Secours Mercy Health

"People will forget what you said, people will forget what you did, but people will never forget how you made them feel. Maya Angelou's words are so true for Amy's Friday emails and her book *Every Storm Runs Out Of Rain*. I felt it. I really felt it, and so will those who lived through the pandemic as close as many of us did."

— Douwe Bergsma, Chief Marketing Officer, Piedmont Healthcare

"Through her insightful and inspiring weekly group emails and her honest and authentic reflections, Amy weaves a compelling picture of the unfolding pandemic in real time and demonstrates the impact of a successful top-tier health system on improving lives and providing hope for their patients, employees, the community at large, and the nation through its leadership and innovation.

It uniquely displays the important contribution of Marketing and Communications professionals to that achievement and the critical role they play in communicating with patients. A must-read for everyone interested in the inner workings of the health care industry through the largest trial it may have ever confronted, or those curious about the intricacies of a positive marketing team impact worthy of emulation."

— Jon Lewin, Emeritus Emory University Executive Vice President for Health Affairs and Emeritus Emory Healthcare President, CEO, and Board Chair, Professor of Radiology, Biomedical Engineering, and Neurosurgery

"Amy Comeau illustrates the importance of one of the most under-appreciated qualities of great leaders - compassion. Amy's weekly emails to her team during the global pandemic is a masterclass on how having the discipline to regularly connect with her employees on a personal level, showing vulnerability, emotional awareness and even some humor, can help get the best out of people and teams during the worst of times."

— Bradley Paskievitch, VP, Legal, DHL Group

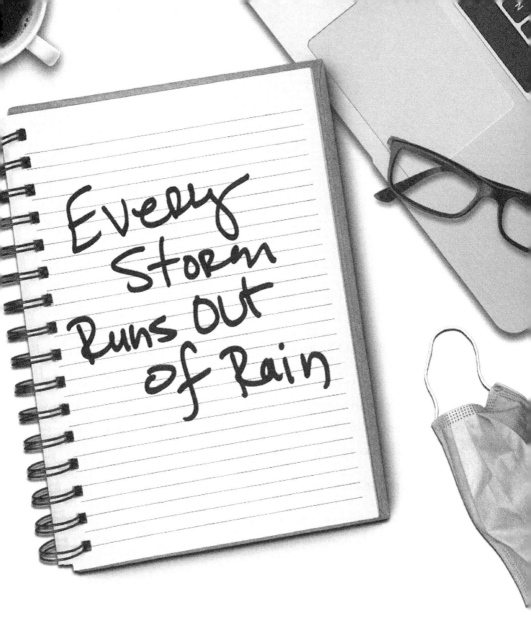

LEADING A HEALTHCARE MARKETING TEAM THROUGH A GLOBAL PANDEMIC

AMY MOUDY COMEAU

"I've found in my life that looking back at the most trying times has helped provide clarity for problems that arise in the present. Amy is doing us all a service by sharing her behind-the-scenes experiences of navigating the pandemic."

— **MATT RYAN**, *Former Pro Quarterback & League MVP*

First printing 2024

Book cover by Amy Moudy Comeau and Andrew Vogel
Book interior by Najdan Mancic

Headshot by Hector Amador, Amador Photo
Photo of Earth Goddess Sculpture by Red Bridge - stock.adobe.com
Photos courtesy of Amy Comeau

ISBN 979-8-9908465-1-7 Paperback
ISBN 979-8-9908465-2-4 Hardback
ISBN 979-8-9908465-0-0 Ebook

Published by Ripples Media
www.ripples.media

Dedication

To my entire family, and most especially my husband Chris and son Josh.

To my marketing team—health care workers and heroes who serve our patients and community.

To all whose lives were impacted by COVID-19, especially those who lost loved ones.

Table of Contents

Foreword

Having lived through the COVID-19 pandemic as both a public health leader and a frontline emergency physician, it's rare for me to want to reflect on the last four years. It's just too painful. Every moment of the pandemic — from the predictable and infuriating PPE shortages, to the unnecessary politicization of life-saving vaccines, to the countless preventable deaths – haunts me.

So when Amy asked me to write the foreword for *Every Storm Runs Out of Rain*, I hesitated. I didn't want to re-enter the psychological space that I had moved beyond. I worried the book would re-open these wounds.

I've known Amy since I was four years old, though. Her family is like a second family to me. Moreover, I had followed her missives to her team on LinkedIn during the pandemic, and (as a health communicator myself) was impressed by her candor and communication skills.

I knew that I had to say yes. And I'm glad I did. When I finally sat down to read her words. . . all I could say was "Thank goodness I did this."

To all of you with the same worries that I had?

Acknowledge your fears, and then put them aside.

Open this book.

Take a deep breath.

And be prepared to be inspired and uplifted.

As a frontline worker, I nodded my head in appreciation at Amy's ability to both encapsulate our experiences and draw universal truths from what her team was seeing. I loved the vignettes about great successes (and felt jealous of Emory's outstanding statistics). I also appreciated the ability to re-live the truths of the early days – unvarnished by the pandemic revisionism that is so rampant right now.

Reading her words of fear, frustration, and hope reminded me that what happened was, actually, real. We didn't imagine it. We were indeed in this together, for a brief and shining moment.

For that, I'm grateful.

Her ability to acknowledge the wide variety of health care heroes – not just clinicians, but housekeeping staff, information technology professionals, public health professionals, and, yes, marketing specialists – is also worth reading, in and of itself. Too often, these days, we think of "health" as being only about the frontline providers. We should all be required to read Amy's words about how the creation of health requires so much more than the clinician!

I loved the book for its leadership lessons, too. Amy's letters to her team exemplify all the best characteristics of a great leader: integrity, clarity, transparency, ability to contextualize. I learned so much about how to manage the unexpected from the way that she wrote to her team.

Her after-the-fact reflections were particularly useful to me (and even inspired me to change a couple of email responses that were sitting in my drafts).

I particularly appreciated how Amy wove her husband and son, her sisters, her parents, and her childhood home into the story – not just because I know them, but because it was a great example of how we (as leaders) are people ourselves! She sets a standard for being a Brene Brown-style leader with a "strong back, soft front, and wild heart."

Every Storm Runs Out of Rain may ostensibly be about the pandemic — but it's much more than that. It's about how to lead with grace through the unpredictable. How to be vulnerable but also clear. How to process change with a team. How to succeed without losing a sense of self.

And, most of all, about how to be human.

Enjoy. I know that I did!

Dr. Megan L. Ranney, MD, MPH
Dean, Yale School of Public Health

Preface

These were times that tested my leadership. Scared and afraid of this virus all around us. The fear of the unknown, but the need to provide calm and strength for my team.

I neglected self-care during this time—adrenaline and a steady drip of wine kept me going. After all, we thought this was an eight-week, work-from-home blip in time. But it wasn't. Eight weeks became eight months, then 18 months and ultimately, a three-year moment in time.

This book began as a "Friday end-of-week" email to my team at the start of the pandemic. Part encouragement, part writing therapy and part ship's log.

I naively thought the pandemic would have a defined start and end, and so would my writing. Now, these Friday emails are here to stay.

As the weeks progressed, my team shared they looked forward to them, and I found I did too. You may find it interesting that I don't have an editorial calendar or plan ahead for them, typically writing them day-of.

One of my lifelong dreams is to become published. As a teenager I wrote poetry and short stories with the hope of writing a book one day.

Fast forward more than 30 years, and I find myself with the privilege of leading an amazing marketing team. The frantic nature of my job and the industries of both health care and marketing took me away from my writing. For several years, I've made it my New Year's resolution to get back to writing. Many a title or idea on my list.

Little did I realize a simple Friday email would reignite my passion for writing. I credit Cheryl Iverson for suggesting I send our "Rise to the Call" print ad to the team—now the first entry of this book. That suggestion sparked a habit I didn't realize I needed, nor my team.

Cheryl and several members of my team suggested I publish these emails as a book. Originally I couldn't imagine why or if anyone would want to publish these. Then, as these things always seem to happen, a fortunate series of encounters and events, catapulted by self-will and some champions, led me to Ripples Media and this very moment.

When I first talked with Ripples founder Jeff Hilimire about if this anthology was publishable, he asked me the question: "Why do you want to publish this book?"

I thought a second and quickly the reasons came flooding out of my mouth:

1. I've always wanted to write a book.

2. To document the pandemic—I don't EVER want to forget how COVID-19 changed our world forever.

3. To help people understand a different, but equally important, kind of front-line health care worker: marketers and communicators, and our non-clinical colleagues that interact with patients daily.

So here we are. It's published! I'm still pinching myself.

The way I see it, there are two ways to read this book:

1. **Read the email entries alone in succession.** Skip the reflections. This will give you a nearly week-by-week account of the pandemic. We literally did not know what was coming next. You can see and feel that from the beginning to the end of this book.

2. **Read it with the reflections** (or, if you picked option 1 go back and read again with the reflections)—these will give you "inside baseball" to what it was like to be a marketer and communicator at the very epicenter of health care during the pandemic.

As you read this book, you'll not only get a nearly weekly recounting of the pandemic (without hindsight); you'll also see through my words, lessons in leadership, self-care, marketing and personal resilience. I hope you'll also see my commitment to my team and my family come shining through. However you read it, thank you.

*Author's Note: While this book recounts my leading my team through a global pandemic, the opinions in this book are purely my own and do not reflect or represent the views of Emory Healthcare or Emory University.

2020

Subject: Can you keep a secret?

Date: Friday, March 20, 2020, 6:55 p.m.

Team,

Can you keep a secret?

I want to share with you that our *Atlanta Journal-Constitution* ad will run as a full page in Sunday's paper. We don't want to scoop ourselves, so please do not forward, post, or share this. We will have ample opportunities to share once it hits homes and newsstands.

As I've mentioned, we have been working with SPM* on a strategic COVID campaign, with a goal to thank our team, our community, and reinforce our expertise. The attached ad is the first asset of the campaign and more will follow in the days and weeks to come.

My thanks to the SPM team for their amazing work, as well as to Chris, Denise, Cheryl, and Larry who provided input today, and to Michelle for helping arrange calendars to get us together. My thanks to Chris, Mark, Mike, Shannon, Maalek, Stef, Tarrance, Tiera and everyone involved in keeping our website, content, and social media updated to inform our patients and help our clinical teams.

To echo the ad, I am in awe. Of all of you. For your support, dedication, flexibility, patience, and understanding this week and on this journey. As Dr. Lewin** has said, we are living through unsettling times with a tough road ahead. And while tough times don't last, dedicated people do.

20

Thank you from the bottom of my heart. Proud to serve as your leader.

Thank you,
Amy

○ REFLECTION

This is my first Friday email to my team. I have Cheryl Iverson to thank for it. Friday, March 20—a week from when then-POTUS declared the COVID-19 pandemic a national emergency.

As I reflect on this time, it seems like weeks passed before we created this "Rise to the Call" ad and subsequent campaign. But clearly it had to be only days. Days! That Monday, March 16 was the last full day of people in the office. My leadership team came in on March 17, St. Patrick's Day, to work through details of how we'd manage a fully remote team for the, ahem, next two months. I'll never forget we all signed work-from-home waivers with return to work dated for June. June! I went home that night to celebrate St. Patrick's Day with my family and raise a toast to this new fun idea of shelter-in-place and working from home.

We ran the full-page *AJC* ad and campaign to thank the community for their outpouring of support. Remember these are the days of people across the globe going out on their balconies at shift change and literally cheering for health care workers everywhere. People were sewing cloth masks, donating hand sanitizer and swim goggles to help protect our teams. It was the epitome of Americans coming

21

together in the face of adversity, when everything in our country (and world) came to a screeching and eerie halt—like Superman trying to turn back time by flying counter-planet spin around the Earth.

*SPM, our agency of record, is now Unlock.

**Jonathan (Jon) Lewin, MD was the CEO of Emory Healthcare throughout the pandemic.

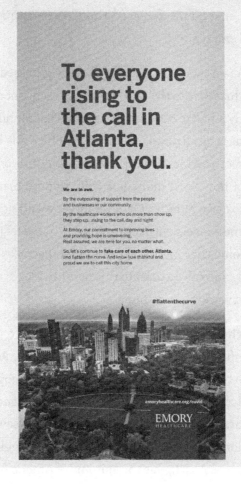

Subject: Thank you

Date: Friday, March 27, 2020, 6:53 p.m.

Team,

Whew! Another week in, and another week closer to getting on the other side of coronavirus.

While this is indeed a marathon, the good news is that marathons do have finish lines. We may not be able to see it yet, but know that with every step, every day, and every week, we get closer to our finish line.

I appreciate how much each and every one of you is stepping in and stepping up to rise to the call. The work we do, that YOU do, matters.

I hope you see and feel how much the community is supporting us. And if you need a reminder, look at the thank you video from the Atlanta Hawks.

Now go get some rest and enjoy this beautiful weather.

Thank you,
Amy

◯ REFLECTION

The beginning of the pandemic was a remarkable and scary time. None of us knew what was happening or quite how to navigate it. Our teams were trying to protect patients and staff while trying to understand a new, fast spreading and deadly virus. Every night at 7 p.m. during shift change, residents in the high rises around our hospitals would come out on their balconies to cheer and thank health care workers. Health care heroes!

If you recall, the NBA had the first major stoppage during the pandemic. If it hadn't felt real yet, the NBA's suspending play cemented that. We later learned that the heartbreaking memorial service for Kobe Bryant became a superspreader event.

Emory Healthcare is the official health care provider of the Atlanta Hawks players and entire organization. While we're technically a sponsor, we've always seen our relationship as a true partnership. This includes the Emory Sports Medicine Complex, which serves as the Hawks' practice facility (Emory Healthcare Courts) and home of basketball operations. It also serves as the official patient care clinic for the general public, who have sports and orthopedic injuries and ailments. Patients and visitors can see the Emory Healthcare Courts and watch live practices from the waiting rooms.

During the pandemic, the "sponsorship" tables turned where the Hawks acted more like sponsors of Emory Healthcare. The video I shared with my team exemplified that. Several

Hawks players recorded selfie videos from their homes which the Hawks then compiled to thank all frontline health care workers (not just Emory) for rising to the call.

The Hawks' support continued when they created the "Feed the Front Lines" effort to support local restaurants and our city's health systems. They also did virtual player visits to keep lifting up our frontline clinical teams.

✉ Subject: Friday Reflections

Date: Friday, April 10, 2020, 8:11 p.m.

Team,

The only way out is through. And just like that, we are a month in, and another week closer to the other side of COVID-19. Dealing with this pandemic is new and challenging for all of us. I know we have our good days and our bad days. That is normal and that is **OK**.

I want to take a moment to share with you two articles that helped frame my own perspective on the emotional stress of this time. I hope you find them insightful as well:

- The first is this *Los Angeles Times*[1] article about our own Dr. Colleen Kraft. While there are many great articles and media stories featuring our experts, I found this one very touching.

- The second is this article from *Harvard Business Review*[2] on Grief. While we are not caregivers on the front lines dealing directly with patients, we are on the front lines communicating with them, providing needed information and supporting our care teams. We are each "grieving" in our own ways, and none are trivial. For me, I'm grieving the loss of watching live sports, eating out at restaurants, and watching Josh perform in band and on the soccer field.

As with every weekend, but especially this one, please take time to unplug, relax, and rejuvenate.

For those who celebrated Passover, are celebrating Easter, or will celebrate Ramadan, I wish you joy and peace in your celebrations.

For those who don't observe, I wish you joy and peace in the ways you celebrate and reflect.

Proud and honored, as always, to have the privilege to lead our team,
Amy

REFLECTION

When life was pulled away from us, at first our Cancer crab tendencies (hard shells, soft hearts) were happy to hermit. But the thought of losing joy in life for an indeterminate amount of time was hard to deal with. My humble family of three are equal parts "experiencers" and "homebodies." At first, we loved the idea of staying home and hunkering down. But when we realized it was more than a mere snow day, we sank.

It was tough. I remember the day we became Atlanta United season ticket holders. It gave me a thrill of arrival like no other. My dad and his colleague, surely at my age, bought season tickets to the Buffalo Sabres and Buffalo Bisons games. I absolutely loved going to these games. As an athlete, I liked to see how they played the game. And decades later I realize the cadence and focus of sports gave me peace. A game with a ball and a stick. Just sit back, watch and follow.

To me, sports are equal parts art and science, like music and medicine. To this day, my male family members make fun of me for always wanting to watch sports. The irony—I'm the mom and the wife and they get tired of my constant desire to escape in sports. I guess I'm the "sports curmudgeon."

As I think back on all of this, the loss of live sports at home and on the TV hit me hard. I hadn't realized how sports had become a meditation for me. The geometry, the chess match, and the mind games; all things I love as a former athlete and current fan.

Subject: TGIF

Date: Friday, April 17, 2020, 7:51 p.m.

All,

TGIF!

I am still reflecting on the amazing and heartfelt 35 minutes of gratitude we spent together during staff meeting this week. There is always a silver lining in the clouds life brings us, and it's clear our silver lining is the jelling as a team we're experiencing.

I'm also grateful, like many of you, to work for Emory Healthcare during this time. I cannot imagine going through this pandemic working for any other organization. I feel fully informed and fully confident in our response and ability to care for our community, today and always. Thank you for everything you do to make EHC great. Please take time this weekend to relax and get away from COVID, the news, and yes, Emory for a bit.

One of my favorite escapes is baking and I hate that I cannot bring goodies in to share with you. In lieu of the real thing, here is one of my favorite brownie recipes that is super easy. Courtesy of Martha Stewart.[3]

Happy baking, happy eating, and happy relaxing!
Amy

✉ Subject: Decompressing with Dolly

Date: Friday, May 1, 2020, 5:12 p.m.

All,

As I sit and reflect on the end of another week during this pandemic, it is hard to fathom that April has already come and gone.

It reminds me of a saying my good friend had about parenthood, especially during the toddler phase: "The days are long, but the year goes by fast." I feel the same way about coronavirus. Many days are long, as are the weeks, but here we are and, all of a sudden, it is May 1!

Last weekend as Dane* and Jon urged the Incident Command Center (ICC) team to find time to relax over the weekend, they asked if we'd send a note with our favorite ways to decompress. I want to share with you what I shared with them. If you feel so inclined, I'd love to hear the same from you. Feel free to drop me a note, snap a photo, or share a meme of your favorite way to unwind.

I'm looking forward to spending some time with Dolly tomorrow (and not having to worry about ICC calls this weekend to boot!).

Have a great weekend and see you on Monday,
Amy

* Dane Peterson was Emory Healthcare's President and COO to whom I reported directly.

From: Comeau, Amy

Jon and Dane,

Even before COVID-19, I liked to walk my neighborhood listening to podcasts to decompress at the end of a long day, with longer weekend walks on the Rockdale PATH trails near our home. My usual podcasts of choice are *Southern Fried Soccer*[4] and *Mouths of the South*; two great podcasts about Atlanta United. We are season ticket holders and going to the games is another great escape for me, my husband, and our 14-year-old son. ATL UTD games are prioritized and cherished family time, so you can imagine we're really missing them not playing!

Since the MLS suspension of play, there haven't been many new episodes to listen to. So, I switched to *Dolly Parton's America*[5]. I found out about it from Maureen Haldeman, during, what I think was, my last in-person lunch before coronavirus changed our daily lives.

She and I were optimistically talking about our upcoming trips. Maureen looking forward to her June trip to Italy, as I eagerly awaited a bucket-list, spring-break trip to Dollywood. We've never been, love roller coasters, and thought it would make a fun family trip, even though we're not country music fans. Maureen had been listening to Dolly Parton's America and recommended it.

I think I started listening to it the weekend after everything started to shut down for COVID-19 and was hooked after the first episode. Now every Saturday, after our 10 a.m. ICC call, I take a long walk around the neighborhood and listen to the next episode. Her story is captivating, and as a former music major, I love the vignettes woven in about ethnomusicology, composition, and history. Yesterday I explored one of my favorite Dolly songs,

"Jolene." Did you know the popular riff from it is written in Dorian mode?

In addition to learning so much about Dolly's life and philosophy, I find it fascinating that the podcast came about because of a friendship Dolly developed with her physician, Naji Abumrad, a surgeon at Vanderbilt. His son, Jad Abumrad, host of Radiolab, begged his dad for an introduction to Dolly, and thus a podcast was born.

I have five more episodes to go, and I'll be curious to see where we are in the world when I'm done with it five weeks from now. Looking forward to a time when we can rebook that trip to Dollywood, though it is hard to envision a world with open amusement parks right now.

Hope you both are having a good weekend and finding time to decompress as well.

Thanks,
Amy

 PRO TIP

In health care, an Incident Command Center is set up to manage crisis situations, like responding to a hurricane, power outage, or other type of disaster. We do mock training sessions to ensure our crisis management protocols are fresh and effective. The arrival of COVID-19 in Georgia prompted the formation of our Incident Command Center. During the height of the pandemic our ICC virtual meetings were twice daily on weekdays and once daily on the weekends. For a span of six weeks, I was on ICC calls literally seven days a week.

◯ REFLECTION

There are many reasons to love Dolly Parton. The icing on the cake for me is her unwavering dedication to science. We know now that Dolly donated $1 million to Vanderbilt University Medical Center to assist with the discovery and development of the Moderna vaccine. Both Vanderbilt and Emory participated in the clinical trials for the vaccine, with Emory serving as the second national testing site. And later, Dolly got her COVID vaccine from Naji Abumrad in a viral video where she also sang her version of Jolene to encourage vaccination: "Vaccine, vaccine, vaciiiiiiiine."

✉️ **Subject: Celebrating National Health Care Week**

Date: Friday, May 15, 2020, 6:16 p.m.

All,

At the end of a different kind of National Health Care Week, I want to express my thanks and gratitude for everything each and every one of you do.

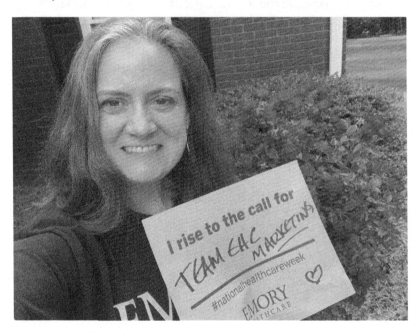

While you may not be clinical caregivers, I sincerely hope you know how much I believe you are frontline health care workers. Everything you do impacts our patients, and, in many ways, our work is the first touch a patient has with Emory Healthcare. You are why I rise to the call every day.

And, if you missed it, here's the amazing GHA (Georgia Hospital Association) "Georgia on My Mind" video[6]. Have a great weekend and see you on Monday,
Amy

🗨 REFLECTION

I had wanted to grow out my gray for a number of years but couldn't figure out how to do it gracefully while sitting in board rooms, meetings, or making presentations.

So, I kept dyeing it. Every. Eight. Weeks. So much money and time invested. My last dye job was early March 2020. This picture was taken about eight weeks later when I should have scheduled my next appointment.

The first "literal" silver lining of the pandemic gave me the chance to finally grow out my gray without judgment. I cannot tell you how liberating this was. I received, at the time, and still get, many compliments on it. It took me about three years to completely grow it all out. I call the journey my "Great Gray Grow Out." At some point, I hope to document in writing and photos the inches grown and what each segment of gray represents which I'd call "These Locks Have a Story."

✉ Subject: Channeling the Dalai Lama

Date: Friday, May 29, 2020, 6:06 p.m.

Team,

Yesterday Ira* shared this "Thought for the Day" from the Dalai Lama on our now twice weekly 5 p.m. ICC Update.

"It is under the greatest adversity that there exists the greatest potential for doing good, both for oneself and for others." — Dalai Lama

How many of you know about His Holiness the Dalai Lama's connection to Emory? I had the great fortune to serve on the communications detail for his 2007 residency. While I didn't get to meet him personally, I got a rare high five from him as he was leaving down the aisle. I was assigned to help manage crowd control and media. I remember that day so clearly. He is inspiring, humble, insightful and has a wicked sense of humor.

So, when Ira shared this quote, not only was I transported to that moment (which brought a smile to my face), I was struck by the meaning of the message. We are under unusual adversity with the COVID-19 pandemic, but as a team, as individuals, and as a system, we are doing incredible good.

My wish for you this weekend is that you continue to thrive on this potential for good and take a moment to reflect on your and our accomplishments over the past 10 weeks. It's truly remarkable.

Thank you for all you do,
Amy

* Ira Horowitz was the Director of the Emory Clinic, and Physician Group President.

 REFLECTION

If you have read *10% Happier[7]*, American journalist Dan Harris' exploration of meditation, you know that Dan Harris was also at this event. He writes about being there and meeting the Dalai Lama in his book too.

✉@ **Subject: Friday Reflections**

Date: Friday, June 5, 2020, 6:34 p.m.

Team,

I don't know about you, but this has been an emotional week—from our continued journey on the coronavirus curve to the protests reminding us how far we still need to go in the fight to end racism.

During this week's Leader Meeting Bryce referenced a quote he heard that goes something like this:

Never would any of us have expected to be experiencing a health pandemic like the world did in 1918, the economics of the Great Depression, and the civil rights movement of the 1960s all at the same time.

Each are historic moments in their own right, and now we're experiencing them all at once. When you add the pervasiveness of social media, fake news and technology, it's almost too much to handle.

And yet, we persevere.

Sharon shared this quote from Abraham Lincoln capturing this perseverance perfectly, not only to the macro-level events, but also to the marketing transformation we are going through.

"We can succeed only by concert. It is not 'can any of us imagine better?' But, 'can we all do better?' The dogmas of the quiet past are inadequate to the stormy present. The occasion is piled high with difficulty, and we must rise with the occasion. As our case is new, so we must think anew, and act anew." — Abraham Lincoln, 1862

I cannot imagine a better work family to have as we go through this time together.

Thank you for all you do,
Amy

✉ **Subject: Poetry**

Date: June 12, 2020, 5:28 p.m.

All,

This week Dr. Bornstein, our Chief Medical Officer, served as our ICC "commander" for the week, and he chose the theme of COVID poetry to close out the calls.

I've saved each in the attached PowerPoint so you can see the faces of two of the poets and get the full impact of how beautifully they are composed. Each one is special and worthy of your read.

Notice the ages of the authors—today's was written by an 11-year-old girl! And the second poem was written by a student who, quite coincidentally, is from the hometown of a physician leader at Emory Johns Creek Hospital.

I found all three to be stunning—a reminder that the pandemic affects all of us, all across the world. It's really remarkable when you step back and think about the collective world experience right now.

As always, I hope you have relaxing and enjoyable weekend,
Amy

- https://www.voicesofyouth.org/blog/poemcovid-19
- https://www.thehindu.com/children/covid-19-poem-will-the-door-ever-open/article31549219.ece
- https://stonesoup.com/post/covid-19-a-poem-of-hope-by-audrey-chuang-11/

✉ Subject: Health Care Marketing Ban

Date: Friday, June 19, 2020, 4:41 p.m.

Team,

Did you know that health care advertising was banned in the United States until 1980? Neither did I.

I discovered this while reading the draft manuscript of our sports ROI project with Goizueta*. David Schweidel, the faculty member we're working with, cited the fact as he described health care marketing.

So, off to Google I went. . ..

Indeed, the American Medical Association banned health care advertising, stating it was unethical in its original 1847 Code of Ethics. This sentiment held for nearly 140 years until the courts overruled the ban as a violation of free speech.

You can read more about this history in Chapter 1 of *Essentials of Health Care Marketing*[8] by Eric Berkowitz. And this article on the early days of hospital marketing by Lauren Strach. According to Berkowitz, Evanston Hospital was the first hospital to hire a dedicated marketing professional in 1975.

For those of you keeping score, Evanston is the home of my alma mater Northwestern University. Ironically Evanston Hospital is not part of Northwestern Medicine, though it was affiliated with Northwestern's School of Medicine for more than 70 years. That relationship came to an end in 2008, otherwise I'd give this historical fact a hearty "Go Cats!"

Staying on the Northwestern connection a bit, I'm sure many of you are familiar with Philip Kotler, often called the father of modern marketing. He introduced the concept of "marketing mix" and is a widely known and published marketing expert. Check out his work, if you haven't already.

For a health care marketing industry that is only 40 years young, I'd say we're doing a pretty darn good job holding our own against our marketing elders in other categories.

And speaking of fathers, I wish all the fathers on our team a very happy and wonderful Father's Day. Thank you for all you do for our team and your families.

Enjoy your weekend,
Amy

Goizueta is Emory's School of Business, named after Coca-Cola CEO Roberto Goizueta.

Subject: Happy Friday

Date: Friday, June 26, 2020, 5:42 p.m.

All,

As we wrap up another busy and productive week, I want to share with you the fruits of our labor.

1. Feel Safe TV Ad, which will start airing next week

2. Feel Safe/Connected Care Radio, in market now

3. Feel Safe/Winship Radio, which will start in rotation in July

4. Atlanta Business Chronicle joint ad with the University in the "A Walk Together" issue today.

5. What to Expect video[9]

And this only scratches the surface! It doesn't cover the emails, the case studies, the blogs, the web work, the Ad Words, the dashboards, the recovery analysis and countless other things on your plates.

Thank you for the tremendous work you all do. I hope you know and feel the difference you make for our organization and in our patients' lives.

Have a wonderful weekend and see you on Monday,
Amy

Q REFLECTION

Gosh, when I see the date and time stamp from this campaign to the previous Rise to the Call campaign, I realize how *close* they are together. The fact that we turned around *two* campaigns in three months is remarkable.

✉ Subject: From surge to surge

Date: Thursday, July 2, 2020, 6:21 p.m.

Team,

It's really hard to believe we are now officially halfway through 2020, and three and a half months into our coronavirus journey. I know many of us hoped we'd be fully on the other side of it by now, although the realists among us probably knew that was a pipe dream.

Truth is, we'll be living with COVID-19 for a while. If you're like me, you may have hit a new slump with this realization and the disappointment with the rising number of cases and hospitalizations across the country, and especially in our own city and state. It certainly hit me hard this week. But there is hope and promise. Let me share a few things that are helping with my own resilience:

1. We are far better prepared for this spike than the one before. We have processes, supplies, knowledge and experience under our belts, that allow us to respond nimbly.

2. We, as a marketing team, are so much stronger than before. Our teamwork and agility are remarkable. Look back to where we were on March 1 and see how much we've accomplished and grown.

3. We have the content. All of the work we have done developing content and messaging for the "Coronavirus Curve" is done. While we may want to create new material and continuously improve upon what we've built, we do not have to start from scratch. The hard work is done, and now we can pivot as needed.

4. We've developed partnerships with our competitors. Let me say that again, we've developed *partnerships with our competitors*. This is truly a public health emergency that impacts our entire industry. I couldn't be prouder of how our systems are coming together to help our community.

5. And then there are the personal things we all do. For me it's walks, wine, talks with friends/family, baking, watching whatever live soccer I can find and trying not to kill my garden. We all have our own ways to escape and recharge, and they are more important now than ever before.

Today Jon Lewin closed out our 5 p.m. ICC call paraphrasing Winston Churchill. "Success is going from surge to surge with optimism and confidence." You are an amazing team and I know we're well equipped to meet this next surge with optimism and confidence. We got this!

Have a wonderful Independence Day weekend and for those of you heading out for longer vacations, enjoy your much deserved and well-earned time off.

Proud to serve our patients alongside you,

Amy

◯ REFLECTION

Was this our first or second surge?

Frankly, I was tired. It was a few days before I went on PTO and furlough. And the fact we were surging, especially before I was going on a much needed break, frustrated me. Not to mention, I was scared about taking my family to red-zone Florida. But as much as I was scared and needed a break, so did my team. They are amazing and we had worked non-stop since the middle of March. They and I both needed this break so much.

Subject: Providing Hope

Date: Friday, July 24, 2020, 5:36 p.m.

Team,

I am glad to be back with my Friday updates and hope you will continue to indulge me with these messages. They've become somewhat of a COVID-19 "ship's log" for me.

When I left work on July 8, Emory Healthcare had a total of 249 patients with coronavirus (C+), an increase of 100 patients in only eight days—150 percent!

Upon my return Monday, we saw another 30% increase to 340 C+ patients, reaching a peak of 352 on Tuesday.

Georgia has seen a 56% increase in cases in the 10 days I was away, the U.S. exceeded four million, and global cases increased 31 percent to more than 15 million.

With numbers like these, it's easy to lose hope.

That's why Dane chose "hope" as his theme for this week's Incident Command Center updates.

Each day he started the meeting with a quote about hope, carefully curated by his executive assistant. I began to write each one down to share with you, but the brisk pace of the meetings left me with half-scribbled quotes in my notebook.

Here are the transcribed quotes from each ICC presentation:

- Monday: "We must accept finite disappointment, but **never lose infinite hope**."—Martin Luther King, Jr.

- Tuesday: "Just as despair can come to one only from human beings, **hope, too, can be given to one only by other human beings**."—Elie Wiesel

- Wednesday: "You may not always have a comfortable life and you will not always be able to solve all the world's problems at once, but don't ever underestimate the importance you can have because history has shown us that **courage can be contagious and hope can take on a life of its own**."—Michelle Obama

- Thursday: "Optimism is the faith that leads to achievement. **Nothing can be done without hope and confidence**."—Helen Keller

- Friday: "**Hope** is the thing with feathers that **perches in the soul** and sings the tunes without the words **and never stops at all**." —Emily Dickinson

Each one speaks to me in a different way, and I've bolded the parts that especially resonated. I hope you will find inspiration, strength, and, yes, **hope** from these too.

Today our C+ patients are down to 298, a 15 percent decrease from our highest peak. See how hope works? I do.

Thank you for all you do to provide hope for each other and for our patients,
Amy

◯ REFLECTION

One of the harder things I had to do during the pandemic was let the team know about our financials. I hadn't had any time off since February 2020. The pandemic took away many weekends, spring break and other times off that you take for granted. Having worked for literally four months straight without a break, I thankfully took my furlough.

I took a week and a half off, using a few days of PTO. Instead of going on our annual Moudy family trip to the Adirondacks. Chris, Josh, and I packed our car and drove to a family condo in Florida for a week, going from Wednesday to Wednesday to avoid weekend traffic.

We had not been out in the world as a family for what felt like years, but really only months. We packed our car full of everything we had in the house: frozen steaks, chicken; fresh veggies; everything so we could avoid going to the grocery store. The YETI cooler did not disappoint!

We stopped once to pee on the trip. I must have made us peanut-butter-and-jelly sandwiches, so we didn't need to go to McDonald's. We stopped at a rest stop, and I put on a medical mask for the first time. Backwards. Didn't even know it until my son said: "Of course you put it on backwards." Me of all people! Fortunately, it was not a big deal.

As we exited the highway and headed to the Key, we observed in real life how some people did not follow the 3Ws (Wear a Mask, Wash Your Hands, Watch Your Distance). People were gathered at the free trolley stops, close together and unmasked. The Daiquiri Deck packed with people. We saw later that the beaches were full of people.

But it was a glorious seven days. We ate great. Grilled out and cooked in. Ordered our first DoorDash—fabulous Thai from a place we should have gone to years before!

We braved the "wild" to pick up Italian from our family favorite, Sardinia. Researched a COVID-friendly pizza place for delivery. And then picking up my birthday dinner from the Lobster Pot.

On my birthday, the doorbell rang—unexpectedly to me. It was a delivery of champagne and a fantastic cake. This was 48 for me. A gift from my parents carefully executed in cahoots with my husband.

In the midst of this trip, I got my Ancestry.com results back. I spent *literally hours* in the deep ancestry hole, finding those I knew were family and trying to make connections. Eventually I traced my mom's side of the family back to the 1400s to Bács-Bodrog, formerly Hungary. And discovered I have roots in a specific part of Sweden.

Knowing I was not allowed at all to connect with or be contacted by work was a welcome and needed respite.

My mind unwound from work (though not completely free from pandemic panic), and I relaxed, slept, laughed and enjoyed time with my family. It was weird, but welcome. And provided the respite I needed to tackle the second half of 2020. (Little did we know there'd be another 12-24 months ahead!)

📧 Subject: Resiliency and Strength

Date: Friday, July 31, 2020, 5:53 p.m.

Team,

Have you ever had one of those days when a word or topic comes up and then you see it everywhere?

Yep, that's been my week. In a good way.

Resiliency and strength are everywhere. It's almost as if the universe is converging to give us all strength. Perhaps it's simply coincidence or perhaps that's perfectly normal for four-plus months into a global pandemic?

Yesterday, in particular, it hit home for me.

First, the *AJC* published John Lewis' "Last Words"[10] to the nation, and earlier in the week his 2014 Emory University Commencement Address was played in the Capitol rotunda as he laid in state. Resiliency and strength come through his words loud and clear. It is still hard for me to imagine Emory, Atlanta and the world without John Lewis.

And shortly after I read his final words last night, I saw the new Nike ad[11]. Nike never disappoints, but this ad is spectacular in every way.

You don't need to be a sports fan to appreciate its impact. And as marketers, we know what it takes to bring this to life. We can marvel at the incredible editing (4,000 hours of footage!), the well-written copy and its simple closing message. The perfect ad. And once again, resilience and strength ring true.

If that weren't enough, yesterday Dane talked about the different muscles we are using and developing as individuals, as a team and as an organization. Noting that we've "learned a lot that will pay dividends into the future" for the benefit of our patients for years to come. We've learned a new and better way of doing things that makes us stronger and more resilient.

And then today Bryce shared this quote:

> *"Life doesn't get easier*
> *or more forgiving,*
> *we get stronger*
> *and more resilient."*

Truer words have never been said. I hope you see and feel our team's resilience, strength, and growth, as much as I do.

We are stronger. We are resilient. We are a team. Thank you for all you do,
Amy

 REFLECTION

John Lewis is simply an icon. Admittedly, I didn't study him like I did Martin Luther King Jr., as a Yankee youth. If he was in my history books in Upstate New York, I don't remember. It was all MLK and Gandhi.

I moved to Atlanta in 1997, thinking I'd just be here for a few years. (Going on 30 now!) Even in the first decade of my time in Atlanta, I didn't realize John Lewis' importance. But I remember seeing him at events (and relatedly, I remember standing in line behind Maynard Jackson at a downtown Starbucks in the early 2000s in stunned awe). I couldn't tell you the moment when I finally understood—deeply understood—not only who John Lewis was, but that he was the everlasting fabric that connected my generation to the Civil Rights movement of the 1960s. John Lewis suffered. He inspired. John Lewis challenged the status quo.

✉ Subject: Gratitude

Date: Friday, August 7, 2020, 5:39 p.m.

Team,

I shared a quick spoiler alert during huddle today, but I want to focus the theme of the week's Friday wrap-up email on gratitude.

Please take five minutes out of your day to watch this incredible *Good Morning America* segment[12] about Tina, Lesa and their amazing teams.

They are the very best example of patient- and family-centered care, leading by example and being brand ambassadors. They provide hope and improve lives as much as our physicians and nurses.

Our 92% COVID-19 survival rate simply could not be achieved without them.

While they may not search for the limelight, they deserve it.

The host's comment at the end, for me, was a stark reminder that gratitude is not always bestowed to every member of the team. It takes a village to do what our health system does every day for our patients. Each and every one of us—from laundry, environmental services, food and nutrition, call center agents, financial services, marketing, communications to the surgeons, nurses and respiratory therapists—plays an important role. Each and every one deserves gratitude and recognition.

Many, many thanks to Lyndsey and Beth for their work on this piece and telling Tina's and Lesa's stories.

Many, many thanks to each of you for the big and little things you do every day to provide hope and improve the lives of our patients.

I'm grateful for all of you,
Amy

◯ REFLECTION

Not all health care heroes are doctors and nurses. They also clean each hospital room and each exam room. Making sure every corner is sanitized, so as not to jeopardize the health of the room's next patient. They are not paid the salary of a physician or a nurse, but their work matters equally. The expert surgical or medical care of a doctor can be undone quickly by an infection. Yes, these are the unsung health care heroes and it brought many of us great joy to see them highlighted and honored on *Good Morning America*.

✉ Subject: You are the Champions

Date: Friday, August 14, 2020, 5:56 p.m.

Team,

This week Sharon led ICC, modeling the week's Resilience theme of "Play". She asked us to send our favorite inspirational lyrics, quotes or poems. Each day she had a song playing as people joined Zoom, included each lyric on the first slide and read them aloud to start the meeting.

We enjoyed some great songs including:

- "What a Wonderful World"—Louis Armstrong
- "Stand By Me"—Ben E. King
- "Feeling Good"—Nina Simone
- "I Can See Clearly Now"—Johnny Nash
- "You've Got a Friend in Me"—Randy Newman
- "Here Comes the Sun"—The Beatles
- Another leader and I both submitted Queen's "We are the Champions" to end the week. I mean, who doesn't love Freddie Mercury?

As I went to look up the lyrics, I came across this incredible video[13] that current day Queen (with Adam Lambert) produced and dedicated to the WHO and HCWs across the world and to raise funds for the COVID-19 relief fund.

A masterful remote performance, coupled with video clips, from back in May. I'm not sure how I missed it then, but glad I found it now.

Take a moment to watch. You'll thank me for the earworm.

If you are so inclined, please send me your favorite inspirational lyrics and I'll share in next Friday's message.

You are the Champions, my friends.

Amy

 PRO TIP

WHO is the common acronym for the World Health Organization. HCWs is shorthand for Health Care Workers.

Every Storm Runs out of Rain

📧 **Subject: A Little Help from My Friends**

Date: Friday, August 21, 2020, 4:38 p.m.

Team,

Sometimes all we need is a little help from our friends.

As we complete the penultimate week of our fiscal year, this couldn't be clearer.

We have so much going on with our own work—the last minute invoice scramble, getting CHUIs out, prepping for MEAC and FY21, visiting Northlake, budget juggling, anticipating flu season, working with our competitors, FEMA grant processing, crunching numbers, managing sports partners, working with the community, writing or designing content, the list goes on and on and on.

There's the work going on around us — students coming back to Emory, caring for COVID and non-COVID patients, onboarding a new university president, testing vaccines and antivirals. . ..

And then our own personal lives, whether it's back-to-school for your kids, worries about your parents, grandparents, siblings, children or grandkids, saying hello or goodbye to beloved pets, moving, paying bills, planning a wedding, even vacationing—it's all a lot to juggle.

So, when Mark sent the classic Beatles song as one of his inspirational lyrics, I was reminded how much we all get by with a little help from each other.

Thank you for everything. And when you feel a little frantic, frenzied or ready to flip, take a breath, remember the amazing support around you and. . . Don't Worry, Be Happy.

Smile and relax this weekend. You all deserve it!
Amy

P.S. Many thanks to Mark for sending in some of his favorite lyrics. If you didn't get a chance to send yours and still want to, please send my way!

 PRO TIP

CHUIs were an acronym for a version of propensity modeling we were using to identify areas at risk for disease. MEAC I earlier described as our Marketing Executive Advisory Committee that was then meeting quarterly. And FEMA: pretty sure everyone knows about FEMA, but those of you not in the health care biz wouldn't know that we had to painstakingly log the hours each member of our team spent on COVID work in order for our system to qualify for much needed FEMA COVID relief funding. I had to carve out at least an hour or two hours a week to research and make sure I had this documented appropriately.

> **REFLECTION**
>
> This was the moment when schools started back in session. Families were given the option to be back in-person but masked, or opt for virtual. It seemed as only five months ago the world shut down for COVID-19, and now suddenly we were hoping for normal. Somehow, we knew things were not yet normal. Especially with the scary flu season upon us.

✉@ Subject: The Sound of Music

Date: Friday, August 28, 2020, 4:49 p.m.

Team,

It's not quite the end of August yet, so Happy New Year's wishes will have to wait until Tuesday's Happy Hour.

I love learning new music and this week Cheryl and Jared shared lyrics with me from two songs I hadn't heard before: "Tin Cup Chalice" by Jimmy Buffet and "Jump" by Madonna.

In a way, they juxtapose the wild ride we've been on since coronavirus changed our lives on March 13. I'm constantly amazed at our team's ability to jump, pivot and blaze the path for Emory Healthcare. Our brand has never been stronger, our patients' experiences ever better, our recovery remarkable—all thanks to the work you are doing.

Enjoy your weekend, may it be filled with great music (new or familiar), sunshine, and warm breezes (hopefully!), a cup filled with your favorite beverage, and maybe even a little Madonna dance party.

Thank you for all you do,
Amy

○ REFLECTION

This marked the beginning of a now annual in-person tradition: Happy Fiscal New Year Celebration! In 2020, we did a virtual happy hour, where I donned a Happy New Year hat and sat in our basement in front of our artificial, but "evergreen" Christmas tree. We leave it up all year long and when I'm feeling adventurous, I decorate it to reflect the current holiday (Valentine's, Halloween, etc.).

Colleagues showed us their pets, their backyards, their bar stash and we laughed. Now, this is an annual in-person event that I schedule for our team, preferably on August 31 but sometimes on September 1, depending on how the days fall.

The past two years we've taken over the bar at a local Italian restaurant near our Northlake office. I buy the first round of drinks and some appetizers on my own personal tab (not Emory's!). We do it from 4 to 6 p.m. to not bleed into the evening hour too much, but also so that it's late enough in the work day to count for happy hour.

It is a time that I cherish. I love seeing how the team engages with each other and the opportunity I have to truly connect individually with my team. I've shared some personal exchanges with unlikely members of the team and those mean the world to me. And, as I've learned, they mean a lot to them too.

Subject: New Year's Resolutions

Date: Friday, September 4, 2020, 5:31 p.m.

Team,

In the frenzy of the final days of each fiscal year, I often forget about, and gladly welcome, the energy that comes with the start of a new fiscal year. I look back on our accomplishments and get excited about the year ahead.

This year is no different. While none of us could have predicted the cards we were dealt in 2020, we did not fold and, in fact, played some of our team's best hands. I'm proud of all we have accomplished together and cannot wait to build upon our success in FY21.

At the start of every fiscal year, I also make my own "new year's" resolutions. Each tailored to the experience and lessons learned from the year before.

Balance is a frequent flyer in them. A global pandemic, shelter-in-place, quarantine, and working remotely certainly have taught us new lessons in striking the right balance in our lives.

And just like we are all unique individuals, so are our needs for balance.

Bryce reminded me of this as he opened each ICC meeting with a reflection on balance, including:

- "There's no such thing as work-life balance. There are work-life choices, and you make them, and they have consequences." —Jack Welch
- "We need to do a better job of putting ourselves higher on our own 'to do' list." —Michelle Obama
- "If you are losing your balance in a yoga pose, reach higher. It will steady you. This is true not just in your practice, but everywhere in your life!"—unknown

The one that struck me the most, however, is Jana Kingsford's quote: "Balance is not something you find, it's something you create."

I remember having a hard time coming to terms with this truth at the height of Ebola and the turn into FY15. I kept yearning for someone to fix my balance, to *give* me balance.

And then I realized: **Balance cannot be given, it is found within.**

So, I made some new fiscal year resolutions to focus on my own balance. And with each passing new year (both fiscal and calendar), I reflect on them. Renew the ones that work and hone others, adapting to the needs at the time.

As we head into the long weekend, please take time to focus on **you**, restore your balance, and, perhaps, make a new fiscal year's resolution of your own.

Happy New Year—here's to a great FY21 ahead!
Amy

✉@ **Subject: Reflecting on 9/11**

Date: Friday, September 11, 2020, 5:52 p.m.

Team,

You may have noticed this is the first year where I haven't asked for a pause during one of our meetings to reflect on the lives lost and lives impacted by 9/11.

This was intentional. Personally, I've been struggling with how to think about September 11th in the midst of a global pandemic.

Nearly 3,000 lives taken from our country in one day by terrorists is a tragedy no nation should have to endure. September 11th changed our country forever. I still think about the lives lost, their families, friends and colleagues, and about the consequential health impact to the survivors near and far, from PTSD to cancer to substance abuse and more. Even 19 years later, the impact lingers.

But here we are. COVID-19 has changed exponentially more lives and it's not done yet. The U.S. has eclipsed 190,000 deaths, with 6,062 Georgians among them. **Our state's lives lost to coronavirus are twice those our nation lost on September 11, 2001.**

You can see how this has been hard for me to reconcile. I'm not sure it is reconcilable.

But then, today Dr. Lewin talked about the work we are doing at Emory to improve lives and provide hope, bringing our 92% COVID-19 survival rate into clear perspective.

We've saved more lives than those that were lost on September 11, 2001. Nearly 4,200 people are reunited with their families, and alive, because they chose Emory.

For that alone I am grateful, and I am honored our team has played an integral part in that positive impact on people's lives.

So tonight, or this weekend, during a quiet moment, take a minute to remember and honor the lives lost and impacted by both September 11 and COVID-19.

Indeed, we should never forget them.

But don't stop there, take a moment to celebrate the survivors. For it is in improving lives that we find hope, and even a bit of joy.

Thank you,
Amy

✉ Subject: Live from the Brandweek Main Stage

Date: Friday, September 18, 2020, 5:59 p.m.

Team,

If you have been on Zoom calls with me during the afternoons this week, you may have found us disrupted by loud club music. As much as I wish I could say that was my playlist running in the background, it wasn't.

It actually signaled the end of that day's Brandweek Masters Live session. (Apparently the mute feature automatically unmutes itself at the close of the Main Stage sessions.)

Sponsored by *AdWeek*, Brandweek is something I've always wanted to attend, but it's been too expensive or came at the wrong time. I was delighted it went all virtual with free passes to the Main Stage for consumer brands. *And yes, we are a consumer brand.*

With an audience of 5,000 marketing leaders from across the globe, Brandweek opened with Marvet Britto interviewing Atlanta Mayor Keisha Lance Bottoms.

Many of us have had the opportunity to hear Mayor Bottoms speak—at the opening of the Emory Proton Therapy Center, or the groundbreaking for the new Winship tower at Emory Midtown, while others have watched her from our homes as she's led the city through the pandemic and social justice protests.

At Brandweek, Mayor Bottoms reflected on our "now normal," her husband's lingering symptoms from COVID-19, and how she encourages her leadership team, saying "we are where we are" to quiet the what-ifs and move forward on progress. She certainly made us ATLiens in attendance proud.

Brandweek continued with marketing leaders from big brands talking about how they had to adjust in the face of COVID-19.

- Dwyane Wade, former basketball star now Chief Culture Officer for CAA (Creative Arts Agency), talked about how important it is to "bring authenticity back to marketing" in order to have a deeper and more loyal relationship with customers. *Sound familiar?*

- Roku's Dan Robbins and Denise Karkos, CMO of SiriusXM and Pandora, talked about how COVID shifted consumer behavior and that two-thirds of Americans (18-34) now stream audio and video when they hadn't pre-COVID. With this shift, they encouraged us all to consider the "Streamer First" marketing plan. *We did that back in the summer.*

- Sumit Singh, CEO of Chewy.com, shared how we need to "be your best in times like these" in order to innovate and advance your brand. *We've certainly done that as a team at Emory.*

- Janey Whiteside, Walmart's EVP for Marketing and Chief Customer Officer, talked about how every member of her Walmart team needs to be storytellers and customer experience officers. That they no longer have time for glitzy ad campaigns and spoke about one of their shining moments creating a how-to video for seniors to learn how to place online and contactless pick up orders. *Sounds a little bit like our how-to videos for Connected Care.*

- And yesterday it was all about Ryan Reynolds. He's quite the personality, slinging around Hollywood zingers like a "cocaine budget" (eek!), but he did share some nuggets that apply to us day-to-day marketers.

The lessons learned from Brandweek apply to all marketers, no matter the industry, service or product. While I learned a lot, there's one thing I didn't need to learn, but Brandweek reinforced: *You are doing industry-leading work.* Even amongst our non-health care peers and the biggest of brands.

Thank you for all you do for keeping our customers first and making Emory Healthcare a brand name.

Have a terrific weekend,
Amy

⬦ REFLECTION

Connected Care was our go-to-market name for our telehealth offering. We had been working on telehealth before the pandemic, doing market research to find a pithier name than Emory Telehealth.

We eventually landed on Connected Care. Our goal for FY20 pre-pandemic was a modest 50 telehealth appointments. But with the pandemic, as well as easing of regulations from the government around billing, coverage and other things, Connected Care became our calling card. It took off like wildfire to the tune of tens of thousands of virtual visits.

✉ Subject: The Apocalypse

Date: Friday, September 25, 2020, 5:46 p.m.

Team,

For this week's recap, I thought I'd share a poem that Dr. Bornstein, our Chief Medical Officer, shared with ICC today. It was written by a Boston ED doctor, Dr. Elizabeth Mitchell, and published by the *New York Times* in March[14].

Titled "The Apocalypse," he warned us the poem was a bit dark, but the reason he shared it was to remind us how far we've come. Commenting that it turns out COVID-19 "was not the apocalypse, nor will it be."

Indeed, what once felt like the apocalypse was not the apocalypse after all. Toilet paper is now on the shelves, PPE in regular supply, kids back in school virtually or in-person and sports are back, and we are all finding our "now normal," to quote Mayor Keisha Lance Bottoms from last week.

It's important to not forget how we felt back in March (even July), but, perhaps even more important, to recognize how far we've come, as a system, as a team, and as individuals, both at work and at home. We are resilient.

Dr. B pointed to the very distinct role we, as health care providers, played in ensuring this wasn't the apocalypse, and the role we play in making sure it won't ever be. I hope this gives you the sense of pride it does me. I'm truly proud of all our team has accomplished in 2020.

Thank YOU for all you do,
Amy

PRO TIP

In the health care industry, we shifted years ago to calling the Emergency Room (ER) to the Emergency Department (ED). ER implies a single room and today's Emergency Departments are true departments with many rooms and many teams committed to triaging and caring for the multitude of patients. EDs were the epicenter of the pandemic.

PPE is shorthand for personal protective equipment, a staple requirement when dealing with infectious disease.

✉️ Subject: 200 Days

Date: Friday, October 2, 2020, 5:38 p.m.

Team,

It has been 200 days since the pandemic changed our world.

203 to be exact.

It's hard to believe, really.

200 days is a long time to be in a transitory state. Some days are good. Some days not so good. And some are a mix of both. For me, today happens to be a "mix of both."

In early COVID, I read and wrote down a quote from Maya Angelou. It sits on the table by my living room chair. Always there. Always a reminder.

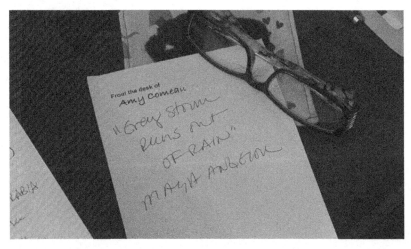

Some days I walk right past it, not giving it or the virus a second thought. Other days the quote gives me a smile, a reminder that we got this.

And some days it draws me in like a trance. I stare at it for a long while, letting the words sink in and gently coax me out of the "coronavirus abyss."

At times, it feels like there's no end in sight. But maybe that's the point? Maybe there's not a "traditional" end. Instead, we adapt. As humans do, as we always do. Yet, I won't lose hope. There will be some sort of end and there will be another side of the pandemic.

So, while we continue to embrace our "now normal," know that this storm, too, shall pass.
Amy

◯ REFLECTION

I wish I could tell you what prompted me to write Maya's quote down on this day. I read a lot of Maya's work in my twenties. In fact, I remember distinctly reading used paperback books of hers when I first moved to Atlanta. I didn't even have a real bed yet. I packed all I could into my modest Saturn and made a real pallet of blankets and quilts in my new apartment, where I slept until I bought a real mattress, frame and box spring—a moving gift from my parents.

I remember spending hours on that pallet reading *I Know Why the Caged Bird Sings* and others of her books. They truly were used, with that soft paper feel that comes from a well-loved book.

Maya Angelou was my first friend in Atlanta. She carried me through long lonely and tough nights of a Yankee girl moving to the Deep South. I am most certain I encountered this quote of hers in my reading back in the late nineties.

✉ **Subject: Relationships**

Date: Friday, October 9, 2020, 5:12 p.m.

Team,

I know we're supposed to avoid talking politics at the office.

But one of Senator Kamala Harris's comments during Wednesday's debate resonated with me, having applications far beyond foreign policy.

She shared Joe Biden's perspective that *"Foreign policy might sound complicated, but really, it's relationships."* She went on to talk about how we all know this from our personal and professional lives.

Often people ask me, "What is the key to success at Emory?" I always talk about the importance of relationships. Developing them, nurturing them, and understanding them. Relationships are—nine times out of ten—the difference between success or failure.

This week I've had conversations with several of you on this very topic. How to navigate roadblocks, see things from the other person's perspective, reach out to someone new, or expand your Emory network. And, in some cases, explaining the nature and dynamics of Emory relationships, not between people, but departments, entities and roles, to provide perspective on a specific challenge.

A favorite quote of mine (and Chuck's wife Terri) is "Change happens at the speed of trust." And that trust is earned (and lost) through the value of our relationships.

I'm proud of the trust and relationships we've built among our team. Keep nurturing them and growing them, so we can continue to be the change we want to see. And don't forget your Emory relationships beyond our department. They are equally as important to create, nurture, and grow.

Now I am going to sign off for a week to focus on nurturing the relationship with my modest family of three. We're looking forward to getting out from behind our work and school computers for a bit, laughing, enjoying the ATL and making unique COVID vacation memories. As Shannon said at our last staff meeting, I too am thankful for PTO and the respite it brings us.

Have a terrific weekend and a wonderful week. See you on the 19th!
Amy

Every Storm Runs Out of Rain

✉ Subject: Finding Beauty All Around You

Date: Friday, October 23, 2020, 5:19 p.m.

Team,

When in the midst of a global pandemic, it's easy to get caught up in the feelings of loss and grief from what no longer is. But in the process of taking something away, of being forced to change our routine, we often find something new.

Something welcome, and even delightful, that we would never have found otherwise.

As some of you know, Chris, Josh and I have a family ritual of visiting Disney during fall break. This October would have been our 10th visit. COVID-19, however, had other ideas and put a halt to our annual tradition. Instead, I attempted to recreate a Disney-esque experience for our Atlanta staycation.

Last Thursday's excursion found us in mixture of EPCOT and the Magic Kingdom with a visit to the Atlanta Botanical Garden. (A perfect outdoor setting to safely follow the 3Ws too!)

It truly is a magical and beautiful place. The "Alice in Wonderland" and "Scarecrows in the Garden" exhibits are what drew us in.

But it was the Earth Goddess who provided my unexpected moment of delight. I could have sat there a long time in the peaceful serenity of her presence and the gently flowing waterfalls surrounding her.

I wouldn't have discovered her—or rediscovered one of Atlanta's hidden gems in the Botanical Garden—had it not been for COVID-19.

So, whether you are a glass half-empty or a glass half-full person, please take a moment this weekend to find and revel in the beauty around you.

And feel free to send me a snapshot of what you find, if you wish. Beauty is in the eye of the beholder, and I'd love to know what delights you.

Happy Friday,
Amy

 PRO TIP

The Atlanta Botanical Garden is a literal hidden gem in our city. Situated adjacent to Piedmont Park and the Piedmont Driving Club, the ABG is an oasis literally in the middle of our city. If I lived in town, I would use my annual membership regularly—as a place to get in my 10,000 steps on the daily.

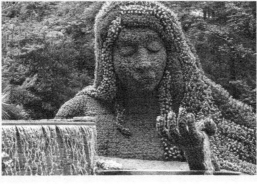

photo by Red Bridge-stock.adobe.com

The Earth Goddess is spectacular. No matter when or what state you see her in, she transfixes and calms. This day, she was being tended to by gardeners. Even still, as you round the corner of the wooded walk, you suddenly happen upon her. People stop and linger, some resting their legs, others gazing as if in a meditative state, while others sketch or point cameras and phones to capture just the right moment.

REFLECTION

I decided not to take my pre-COVID-approved spring break time off. It was the first week in April, we were in lockdown and there was too much work to do. I had early-pandemic stamina, adrenaline, and energy. When I had to take furlough in July, I realized just how much time off was needed. So, when Josh's fall break came around, I took the whole week off.

Sad the pandemic kept us from our annual Disney trip, I set out to make the week a "Disney at Home" vacay. I bought beach-scented candles for our home to recreate the signature smell at Disney's Beach and Yacht Club where we'd stayed the past several years, and a Mickey waffle maker to replicate Chef Mickey's famous Mickey waffles.

Monday—(Hollywood Studios day at Six Flags Over Georgia)—Six Flags was open for Columbus Day and Fright Fest. We took a big gamble, but after checking their COVID protocols and having comfort we were outside and masked, we went. It was weird, but so much fun. The screaming—albeit masked—on the roller coasters was a balm for our souls. I don't think we realized how much we needed that release.

Tuesday we emulated the now defunct Disney ESPN Zone with Josh's club soccer team playing outdoors.

Wednesday—(Animal Kingdom day at Zoo Atlanta). Zoo Atlanta is another amazing spot in Atlanta. And great place to get steps in if you live nearby and can go regularly. I'm pretty sure Josh and I even got on the carousel.

Thursday—(Epcot and Magic Kingdom day at Atlanta Botanical Garden) On this day, *Alice in Wonderland* met Fantasyland and the Mad Hatter's Tea Cups of Magic Kingdom, where the Garden felt much like my favorite "Living with the Land" boat ride at EPCOT. Josh hates that ride, but I LOVE seeing the living garden and what they're growing, and the hidden Mickeys.

Friday—(Mini-golf at Pirate's Cove)—Traveling from Rockdale County to Gwinnett County was a haul for Josh and me, but it was worth it. I found a random specialty hot dog place in the middle of nowhere on the way there. Really in the middle of nowhere.

When we got there, I almost worried about what I had done, but it was delicious. Ordering at the window, I brought the hot dogs, fries and drinks back to the car. We sat in the driver and passenger seats enjoying them at a random industrial park. Mimicking Fantasia mini-golf and hot dogs on the Boardwalk.

It was a fun staycation, and a reminder that there really is beauty all around you—if you just seek it out.

✉ Subject: The best is yet to come

Date: Friday, October 30, 2020, 4:16 p.m.

Team,

I want to say how incredibly proud I am of all of you. I know we mentioned it during Huddle this morning, but last night's Marketing Executive Advisory Committee meeting was nothing short of spectacular.

Nearly 10 years ago, I had a vision of what a CRM (Customer Relationship Management platform) could do for Emory Healthcare. I remember sitting in the basement swing space at Emory Saint Joseph's Hospital on a conference call with Nick from MedSeek. He and his colleagues talked with me about the promise of propensity modeling, personalization, better targeting, and using control groups for more effective marketing. It seemed an impossible dream to bring that to Emory.

A little more than 10 years before that call, I had the unique opportunity to take part in New Employee Orientation at the Ritz-Carlton Atlanta. I wasn't working there, but the Managing Director of the Atlanta Opera (where I was working) knew the hotel's leadership team. After two unusual events threw our opera company into crisis mode, Alfred asked if several of our staff could sit in on the session to learn more about the Ritz-Carlton's legendary service promise and training.

It was there, in a tiny, staff conference room tucked away in the recesses of the hotel on Ellis Street, that I truly first learned about customer relationship management. They didn't have Salesforce (eventually created in 1999). Instead, they used a fascinating and complex system of index cards—yes index cards—to note customer preferences, such as down pillows or blue M&Ms.

The Ritz taught me to stop saying "No Problem" because in the mere fact of saying "no problem," you imply there was a problem to begin with and put the other person on the defensive. Instead, I started saying "my pleasure." I also learned to stop pointing when people ask for directions and instead walk them to their destination or to another human who can help. I still do this today at Emory Healthcare, helping our patients and families get from Point A to Point B in our complex maze of bridges, hallways, and buildings.

Then and now, I knew marketing had a major role to play in transforming how Emory Healthcare interacts with our customers. But there was a lot of transformation that needed to happen within our organization and our team to bring that to life.

So, last night, when all the pieces and progress came together—from Content to Community Engagement to CRM—it was like winning the World Series or the Oscar for Best Picture. I was, and still am, over the moon with pride.

This is a true inflection point for our team, for Emory Healthcare, and for our customers and patients. Remember it, reflect on it, and celebrate it.

And while this feels pretty great, I know the best is yet to come.

Thank you and have a wonderful weekend,
Amy

PRO TIP

CRM stands for Customer Relationship Management. In this instance, CRM is a technology tool that marketers in all industries use—or aspire to use—to manage their customer database. If you've received a personalized message from any brand—be it Starbucks or Hilton—they've used a CRM system.

Implementing CRM has been a lifelong career goal of mine dating back to the late 1990s. Finally, it came true in fall of 2019 when we signed the contract for our first CRM at Emory Healthcare. Little did we know how handy it would come in with the global pandemic around the corner!

MEAC stands for Marketing Executive Advisory Committee. This is a group of stakeholders I convened when I first stepped into my leadership role nearly a decade ago. It helped provide transparency and shared decision-making to advise our executive team on marketing strategies, initiatives, and budgets. It comprised hospital CEOs, physicians, and administrative leaders of our signature service lines, and other key business unit leaders.

✉ **Subject: Peace**

Date: Friday, November 6, 2020, 4:41 p.m.

Team,

It's been quite the week.

In conversations with several of you, we touched on a general feeling of anxiety, for many myriad reasons.

It's no surprise. Pandemic fatigue. Election uncertainty. A time change. Marketing plans. Goals. Year-end reviews. Power outages. Unexpected twists and turns. Even the holidays. It's a lot.

It's easy to let it overwhelm. But then I came across this quote last night:

> *peace.*
> *it does not mean to be in a place*
> *where there is no noise, trouble*
> *or hard work. it means to be in*
> *the midst of those things and still*
> *be calm in your heart.*

And — at the risk of dating myself yet again — it reminded me of the end of the *Wizard of Oz* when Glinda the Good Witch told Dorothy she had the power all along, she just had to learn it for herself.

Please take time this weekend to rest, relax and use your own power to find the calmness in your heart.

Happy Friday,
Amy

✉ Subject: Friday the 13th

Date: Friday, November 13, 2020, 6:00 p.m.

Team,

For today's theme, I chose the unusual and much feared *Friday the 13th*.

And I have a confession. I **LOVE** Friday the 13th. I love **#13**.

My birthdate is a **13**. So, I never understood the superstition that burdened the number 13. Did it mean I would be forever unlucky because I was born on the 13th?

Why didn't hotels have a 13th floor? Didn't people realize the 14th floor was really number 13 anyway? And, what was so horrible about the 13th on a Friday?

I actually felt bad for the number 13.

Instead, I embraced it. Proudly defended it. Appreciated its beauty and simplicity. A perfect prime number after all!

13 is my favorite number.

I chose it whenever I could as my jersey number playing sports. I still get excited when I see it proudly used and worn. I see you Ronald Acuña, Jr. and Alex Morgan… It's my go-to number the rare times I play the lottery or roulette.

I especially look forward to the years my birthday falls on Friday the 13th. It's cause for extra celebration. I was ecstatic when my 40th fell on Friday the 13th. It seemed so apropos. Even threw some epic Friday the 13th birthday parties when I was a kid.

While I'm not a Jason fan, the date did give us a whole series of iconic horror movies. As well as the classic campy movie, *Saturday the 14th*. My sisters and I loved that one. Check it out if you haven't, it's another 1980s classic.

So, don't let Friday the 13th get you down. Instead consider it a rare gem worth celebrating, like I do. Go enjoy the remaining hours of this Friday the 13th, in this crazy year of 2020, and have a terrific weekend.

Thanks for all you do,
Amy

✉️ **Subject: Thanksgiving**

Date: Friday, November 20, 2020, 5:05 p.m.

Team,

As folks begin departing for Thanksgiving, I want to take this moment to share how very thankful I am for all of you.

2020 has tested us all and we still have six weeks to go (wow—only six weeks!). Many have spoken of the "pandemic fatigue" that we just can't seem to shake, requiring us to dig deeper into our resolve, to hunker down for the winter and get through this next phase of our COVID-19 journey.

The good news is there's finally a light at the end of the tunnel. Just how long that tunnel is, we're not certain, but the end is clearly lit now.

I hope you share the pride I have in knowing that Emory is a major part of bringing that light to life. Our vaccine and therapeutics trials. Our 92% survival rate. Our continued dedication to improving lives and providing hope. All reasons to shine brightly.

This Thanksgiving comes at the perfect time. A time for us all to take a break. A time to focus on family and friends, with new and creative ways to safely celebrate together. And, most importantly, a time to focus on ourselves. Please take this time to rest, relax and restore yourselves.

My very heartfelt thanks for each and every one of you. Happy Thanksgiving,
Amy

Every Storm Runs Out of Rain

⬭ REFLECTION

With the passage of time, I remember this as one of my favorite Thanksgivings, but man, was it fraught with stress.

My family missed each other. We all wanted to see each other. We all had different tolerances for exposure. But we all agreed we did not want to put our parents and Chris' parents at risk. There were tense texts and a stressful sister family Zoom with the brother-in-laws chiming in.

Because I work in health care, I was more strict than everyone. For one, I had to be, because of what we were taught and expected to do at work. But also, I knew more, and I saw and heard on the daily about those who were in the ICU, on the brink of death. Those who made it and those who did not. I didn't want to be the catalyst for a death or a superspreader in my family.

For my sister and her family in DC, it was an easy decision not to come. It would be a long drive with a toddler and not worth the drive or the exposure risk. But for my sister and her family in Ohio, the decision was harder. I wanted them to come, but only if they quarantined. Given their circumstances with kids in school and their own pandemic circles, they couldn't pull it off. My sister and I decided it was best for them not to come, no matter how badly we wanted to see each other, again because we didn't want to put Mom and Dad nor my in-laws at risk. It was a tough, tough call, but in the end, I still believe it was the right decision.

For our Thanksgiving, with us 3, my parents and in-laws we did everything outdoors and it was spectacular. Fortunately, the weather cooperated. We used our pop-up catering tent and put out six-foot tables for each family. I made single-serve appetizers so we could still enjoy cocktail hour without cross-contamination.

Chris and I cooked. I made my first-ever homemade soup, a fennel celeriac recipe, using newfound produce from Misfits Market. (Misfits Market is an online grocery store dedicated to eliminating food waste.)

We did have all the fixings inside as a buffet, but each family went in one-by-one, like a buffet wedding. As the evening went on, Chris brought out his Solo stove and we enjoyed wine, laughs and desserts by the fire.

To this day, I have wanted to recreate the outdoor Thanksgiving, but alas, the weather has not been conducive. Perhaps that's meant to be. Another pandemic silver lining. A fantastic memory in a desperate time. And thankfully we're all still standing.

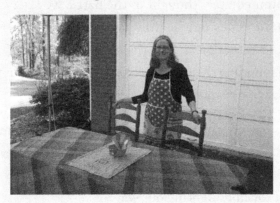

✉ Subject: Light a candle

Date: Friday, December 11, 2020, 5:33 p.m.

Team,

Last night Hanukkah began, with menorah candles lighting windows and homes around the world.

Though I am not Jewish, I have found beauty in Jewish holidays, traditions and music. I especially enjoyed my best friend's daughter's bat mitzvah via Zoom earlier this year.

Many of you know the story behind Hanukkah, so I won't retell it. However, as I was reading more about it today, I came across this message on its meaning from Chabad.org:

"Never be afraid to stand up for what's right. Judah Maccabee and his band faced daunting odds, but that didn't stop them. With a prayer on their lips and faith in their heart, they entered the battle of their lives—and won. We can do the same."

Sounds eerily familiar, doesn't it?

For me, I immediately thought of the battle we are facing with COVID-19. At times our health care industry—our front-line workers, our researchers, and the supporting cast of so many, like us, surrounding them—feels like we are facing daunting odds and racing against an ever faster ticking clock.

None of us has ever faced a pandemic before. As a humanity we are in the battle of our lives. Yet with confidence, perseverance, a little hope and a lot of science, we will get through this, with the promise of vaccines lighting our way.

So, to those of you on our team who celebrate, a heartfelt Happy Hanukkah to you and your families.

And to all of you, remember you are the light that makes our team so bright.

Thank you for the role each of you play in our continued battle against coronavirus. You are improving lives and providing hope every day.

Thank you,
Amy

 PRO TIP

If you've noticed I weave the phrase "Improving Lives and Providing Hope" into many of these messages, you're right. It is Emory Healthcare's True North statement. Not our tag line, but a reminder of our core purpose, mission, vision and values.

✉ Subject: Simple Gifts

Date: Friday, December 18, 2020, 5:58 p.m.

Team,

What a week.

The hope that we've been waiting for since March 13 has finally arrived, and it is bringing joy to so many health care workers across our country. And, what an incredible honor it is to be part of world history. I get emotional every time I think about it.

It's really hard to put it into words, and every time I try, instead of words, I hear music. Simple Gifts to be exact.

I'm sure you all are familiar with the Shaker tune. *"Tis a gift to be simple, tis a gift to be free. . ."*

It has been a favorite of mine for a long time. I remember studying it in music school when learning how Aaron Copeland quoted the tune in his famous *Appalachian Spring*. Our bridesmaids and groomsmen walked down the aisle to a brass quintet playing it at our wedding. I even referenced Simple Gifts in a blog I wrote for Emory Healthcare describing my experience delivering gifts on behalf of our marketing team to the Winship Cancer patient family we adopted, many years ago.

The vaccine truly is a simple gift. A gift to the world, full of hope, science, protection and promise.

And while we have a bit to wait before we can receive ours, I hope you find the same joy and pride I do, in knowing we are part of that gift coming to life.

So, as you all embark on your holiday breaks over the next days and week, I hope you will enjoy the simple gifts around you. Whether it's a silly box of Cheeto's Mac 'n Cheese, time with family, a good book, a walk with the dog, or the time to take a nap, I hope your holidays are filled with simple gifts that bring you joy.

Thank you for all you do,
Amy

⟲ REFLECTION

I first questioned whether I was a true health care worker with the vaccine distribution categories, so did my team. This is both true and unfortunate.

We are not clinical care providers, yet we work at a health care institution—does that not make us health care workers? But according to the criteria, we did not technically qualify for the first round of vaccination. They were reserved, as they should have been, for those most vulnerable to the virus— those providing direct clinical care. Frontline staff became synonymous with clinical care providers, but the truth is they cannot do their work without the non-clinical health care workers. It takes all of us.

Burnout in health care is real. And it is not isolated only to the doctors and nurses. The attention on burnout goes to the obvious. I am not doubting that, nor discounting it. Their experience is real.

And so is ours.

Burnout comes in many forms. The obvious and the not-so-obvious. Both matter and both should be recognized and addressed.

Yet, in spite of that, to feel that I am a less-than health care worker in a once-in-a-lifetime global pandemic is soul crushing. It took uploading a photo of my work ID to qualify for a health-care-worker online shopping discount (with MARKETING clearly marked on the badge) to realize that yes, indeed, I am a health care worker.

One of the reasons I wrote this book is to share the story of the unseen and unexpected frontline workers—health care marketers and communicators, as well as our brethren in finance, IT, operations and planning.

2021

✉️ **Subject: Hello 2021**

Date: Friday, January 8, 2021, 4:58 p.m.

Team,

So... 2021 came in with a bang, didn't it?

A runoff election, a siege on our Capitol, the depths of the third surge, two days of planning sessions and, oh yeah, preparing to start vaccinating our patients!

It has been the craziest start to a new year ever. But, for me, the vaccination work is perhaps the most important work I've done in my life. Ever.

The work we are doing truly is lifesaving. I'll say that again. The work YOU are doing is LIFESAVING.

Every person vaccinated is a step against this deadly virus. A step toward our future. A step toward a moment Dr. B. shared on ICC this morning:

"One day this is going to be over—can you imagine that day? How we'll come out into the sun and laugh and hug and sing and dance and hold hands? I'm living for that day. It'll be like nothing we've experienced before."—Glennon Doyle, *One Day This Is Going to Be Over*

I know we are all living for that day. In fact, we are all literally working to make that day happen.

So, when the work, the chaos, the weight of it all feels too much, remember this: You are critical to saving lives. You play a role in helping the world ultimately celebrate in the sun.

That will be a glorious day.

Thank you,
Amy

 REFLECTION

Every time I read this email and sit to write a reflection, I can't. There is SO MUCH wrapped up in this moment in time. Like a strange, and unwanted, ever-lasting-gobstopper.

My first reaction, reading this again three years later in early January 2024, is that Glennon was wrong. That day never happened. There was no singing and hugging and dancing in the sun.

The siege on the Capitol—surreal, unreal, and yet, real. Sadly, real. A horrible, sad and scary time for our country and our democracy. And it happened on top of so much stress. People were dying from coronavirus. Vaccines, while finally available, were not widespread so it created a time of haves and have-nots.

I remember people literally driving hours from Atlanta to Savannah to get their first dose, while others, literally, heckling my team through email responses and viral social media about the poison of vaccines.

It was the first in time I realized that workplace violence could come through the written word. The emails, DMs, and social media comments my team had to field from anti-vaxxers were verbally offensive and violent. "You can take your 'GD' vaccine and shove it where the sun don't shine" was one of the milder ones from someone who met the criteria for early vaccination! All the while, most of my team did not even yet qualify for, but desperately wanted, the vaccine.

✉ Subject: There is a balm

Date: Friday, January 15, 2021, 6:50 p.m.

Team,

Yesterday I thought I'd get a head start on this email, knowing I'd be at the Vaccine Clinic all day today, and it was tough.

If I may be frank, it has been an exhausting week, and I couldn't find the right words to say. I had a long draft about grace and patience with each other, other colleagues, and our patients. All important messages, but it rang hollow.

But then I spent today checking in cars and employees at the Northlake vaccine drive-through clinic, and now my words come easily.

My legs are tired, my face sunburned, but my heart full. So very full.

To see the excitement and hear the heartfelt gratitude from each person coming through was exactly the balm I needed. A reminder of the important, life-saving work we are doing. Of the incredible impact Emory Healthcare has on our community.

I understand my feelings mirror those that worked last night's pilot with patient vaccinations. This morning, our Chief of Emergency Medicine said "The kudos from the patients last night was unbelievable!" And I continue to hear so many similar stories.

If you have not had a chance to experience this incredible connection to our work, I encourage you to continue to sign up for shifts to support the vaccine clinic. It may be just the balm you need too. I know I will be back again.

And, we cannot let the week go by without celebrating that we vaccinated our first patients!! What a milestone! You made that happen.

So, at the end of a long, but historic, week, I share with you a heartfelt thank you from Dr. Lewin during a Zoom call just now to a small group of leaders whose teams have been instrumental in our patient vaccination efforts. (This means YOU.)

"What you all have done is so amazing, really beyond words. I cannot possibly say how grateful I am for all you have done. Thank you so much for doing that."

Thank you for continuing to improve lives and provide hope,
Amy

🔍 REFLECTION

I remember this day well. This week, and the previous one, were draining — not to mention the previous 10 months of pandemic life.

We began vaccinating actual patients using an old Sears Automotive drive-thru location. Lines of cars coming though. I stood on my feet for several hours, in what I call "ski sun" (cold but sunny enough to get both windburned and sunburned) and it felt so good. I checked email confirmations and handed out vaccine cards to hundreds of happy, giddy, thankful and nervous people. Our first opportunity to offer mass vaccinations to our eligible patients.

These patients would not have been in line if it were not for the efforts of my team. We used our marketing automation and CRM system to allow patients to request a vaccination. When their criteria met the government's criteria for vaccination, we emailed and texted them. This was complex data work that only my team could do given the limitations of our EMR (electronic medical records). The patients I helped in line that day would not be there without marketers invisible and invaluable frontline workers.

✉ Subject: Do you see what I see?

Date: Friday, January 22, 2021, 5:54 p.m.

Team,

What a difference two weeks make. Take a minute to look at these slides:

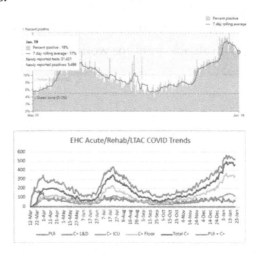

Do you see what I see? While numbers are still high, I'm breathing a sigh of relief today that hopefully we've passed the apex of this third wave.

We are all thankful to see the numbers dropping. Today our ICU/CCU units reported their numbers have dropped from a record high of 152 C+ patients two weeks ago to 115 today. Our EDs reported that ILIs are now in the 30s percentage range, down from highs in the 40s and 50s earlier this week.

While the pandemic is far from over, we can take some relief that this recent surge appears to be on the downward trajectory.

Closer to home, these first three weeks of January have been a whirlwind and a roller coaster when it comes to vaccinating our patients.

While we await news of a more consistent vaccine supply chain, we should all take a moment to celebrate the fact that Emory Healthcare has completed nearly 30,000 vaccinations to date. Thirty thousand!

That is an amazing accomplishment and one of which you should be proud. YOU made this happen.

Whether you wrote copy, updated the website, programmed data, built a form, proofread, supported a teammate, worked a shift at the clinic, or got the vaccine yourself, you are a major contributor to our accomplishment of 30,000 vaccinations. And this is only the beginning. . .

As always, THANK YOU for all you are doing for our team and for Emory Healthcare. Each of you plays an important role in the work that we do, whether it is COVID-related or our standard marketing work. All of it is important, as are each of you.

I hope you each find time to rest and relax this weekend. You deserve it.

Thank you,
Amy

 PRO TIP

ILIs are Influenza-Like Illnesses. I had been working in health care for 15 years and it took a pandemic for me to hear that acronym. The first time I heard it in 2020, I had to look it up. Embarrassed to ask what it meant, especially on an incident command call.

ICU = Intensive Care Unit

CCU = Critical Care Unit

C+ became our shorthand for COVID Positive.

◯ REFLECTION

Frankly, this week pissed me off. Working nearly 24-7 since mid-March 2020 and finally the joy of vaccines and vaccinations upon us. A light at the end of the tunnel. And whammo—a government shortage of vaccines.

During this week, I had a Zoom meeting with colleagues about vaccine distribution, changes in eligibility and availability, that went until eight in the evening. And I woke up talking to the same women at seven the next morning on the same topic.

I remember making the joke: "Ladies, I feel like I slept with you all night." It was an awkward joke but rang so true. After all we had been through, with the vaccine and the promise of hope of life after COVID—and as soon as we figured out how to distribute it efficiently—the government had a shortage. Add in the beginning of many frustrating, but understandable, qualifications for vaccination with frequent changes that caused us to rework our processes each time. We were exhausted.

✉ Subject: Impermanence is the only permanence

Date: Friday, January 29, 2021, 6:19 p.m.

Team,

At the risk of sharing too much and inviting hippie jokes upon myself, I'm going to confess that I started meditation this year. Tried it a couple times in 2020 but couldn't find the discipline to get it going.

Then a colleague shared a 30-day trial of the Calm app with me. Truth be told, he shared it with me back before Thanksgiving, but, alas, I felt too busy to bother with it.

But after the frenzied start to 2021, I decided to give it a try. For the past week and a half, I've started each work day with the "Daily Calm." This 10-minutes-a-day has earned a regular spot in my resilience routine.

I am not here to sell you the benefits of meditation. Instead, I want to share with you the message from one of this week's sessions that really spoke to me.

It's this concept of "impermanence."

- **Impermanence. The idea that nothing lasts forever.**
- **Essentially the only thing permanent in this world is impermanence.**

Tamara Levitt, who narrated the session, went on to say: "This lesson [of impermanence] is contrary to human nature. Our instinct is to resist change...But impermanence is an unavoidable law of nature. The more we resist change, the more difficult we make our lives."

Instead, she says, we should focus on experiencing things as fully as we can as they happen and then gracefully let them go as they naturally come to an end.

So, while her point was more about resisting aging, not wanting kids to grow up so fast, or getting out of bad relationships, I immediately connected to our lives today, and the battle that is coronavirus.

While we are perhaps experiencing this pandemic more fully than we would like, there is a peace in knowing that this too shall pass. We don't know when, but we can be certain it will be impermanent.

Until then, please use this weekend to engage in your own preferred methods of resilience and find time to fully experience and enjoy the things that bring you joy.

Thank you for all you do,
Amy

REFLECTION

The panic attacks. This was not my first of the pandemic. I was cleaning my guest-room-turned-office to set up my new stand-up workstation. I was dusting and cleaning and suddenly felt a pain in my arm and became breathless. I worried I might be having a heart attack. I got dizzy. I felt like I was going to throw up. The panic attack worsened because I knew ALL of our EDs were full with long wait times. I didn't know how to ask for help at work to get me in ASAP or if I even needed to go to the ED. So my head and body swirled and swirled.

I went on to have four or five panic attacks within the span of two weeks. One was set off by a funny feeling in my leg, and I immediately worried it was a blood clot or aneurysm that would find its way to my brain. This panic attack evolved into a series of repeated episodes while I tried to sleep. Understand this: I have had maybe two or three panic attacks before in my entire life. All of a sudden, I had four or five in the span of two weeks. One hit me in the middle of our weekly team meeting while I was calmly detailing to my team the latest with vaccine distribution changes. I felt like I was going to faint—while speaking via Zoom to my team! I had 30 minutes after that meeting to calm myself before having to be lucid and focused for a noon meeting with our CEO and executive team about how we'd tackle vaccine communications.

Until that point, most of my panic attacks happened after hours, not during the work day. This was the first one that happened during work, and it spooked me. So much so that I texted my boss about it. He was immediately responsive, which I appreciated, and called me right after that big meeting.

He suggested I text my physician. I didn't have his number, but he did. I texted my primary care physician (PCP) and he got me in for a visit the very next day.

I didn't share any of this with my team, but it is the reason I started meditation.

✉ Subject: Kindness

Date: Friday, February 5, 2021

Team,

As I reflect on the week—really the first five weeks of 2021—I want to talk a bit about kindness.

It is clear that in addition to a shortage of vaccine, the world around us is experiencing a shortage of patience and kindness.

We've had our fair share ourselves. Whether it's the "take your vaccine and shove it" responses to email or social, our call center teammates taking heat from angry customers, or criticism from frustrated internal clients (read: physicians), it doesn't feel good to be on the receiving end of negativity.

People forget there are human beings on the other side of emails, phone calls, and social comments.

While we often hear and see the negative, it is important that you know how many people are grateful and thankful for the work you are doing.

Here are just a few comments from grateful patients this week:

- *A competitor ". . .sent me a message via MyChart saying essentially, 'don't call us, we'll call you' when you are eligible. Not patient-friendly and **not nearly as informative or communicative as Emory has been** by any extent."*

- *"A friend and my wife who are Emory patients have requested and received vaccinations at the Northlake Mall site. **They registered at the Emory website.** She is a caregiver; he is in his seventies. **The site was very efficiently run.**"*

- *"I called everyone and they all put us on waiting lists, but **Emory came through. . ."***

- *"Getting my first shot from Emory Healthcare tomorrow after being on the waiting list for a while. **They came through!**"*

- *"Hello, I wanted to let you know how amazed I was this morning with the efficiency, patient care, and helpfulness of all the staff at the Northlake Mall site. My appointment was scheduled for 8:45 am and I was home by 10:00. After seeing the stories on the news about long waits, standing in lines, and having to travel far, my experience today was outstanding.*

- ***If it weren't for being able to register on Emory's site, I know I would not have received the vaccine for weeks.** Like many others, I had no success with the county sites, Publix, or Kroger. When I received a message. . .and was scheduled today, it was an unexpected surprise. **Emory is to be congratulated on a job well done and for their amazing staff.**"*

I hope you can see the kindness and appreciation in their comments. Kindness truly is a virtue. **You** make all the difference for our team, each other and our patients.

Thank you for all you do,
Amy

⊙ REFLECTION

This was another stark reminder that my team experienced workplace violence. In health care, workplace violence is described in four types. We take annual learning courses each year, a requirement, to identify and report workplace violence. An unwelcome result of the increase of gun violence in our country. Written or verbal threats are one type of workplace violence.

My team, who sent the emails out about vaccines, got far too many responses from anti-vaxxers that were plain old mean and nasty, often vulgar and using foul language. I mean, what makes someone so mad about a voluntary vaccine that they have to lash out at their health system for offering it to them? Think twice before you lash out at someone—you have no idea what they are going through.

I also remember starkly a nastygram we got that week that made my team feel unappreciated. There is so much work, art and science that goes into marketing and it hurt to receive a snap response of dissatisfaction on a piece of creative.

I also had folks on my team not getting along—which made leadership even more challenging, especially given previously noted panic attacks and personal health care concerns.

All of this together inspired my email to the team on kindness.

✉ **Subject: A Super Bowl of Ads**

Date: Friday, February 12, 2021, 5:39 p.m.

Team,

As we wrap up this week, I want to take a minute to reflect on the Super Bowl. Not the game itself, but the advertising showcase that it is.

AdWeek's content focused solely on Super Bowl commercial coverage this week. Focusing, as always, on the winners and losers, as well as LOTS of talk about the absence of masks in the ads. Did they forget we are in a global pandemic?

My personal favorite ad is "Drake from State Farm."

I love how State Farm has evolved its brand over the years. Never straying from their core brand elements in Jake, their motto and their advertising model. They've done a wonderful job staying connected with their consumers, relating to their target audiences and integrating humor, celebrities, concepts and, yes, branding in their ads.

There is not a chance you won't remember State Farm as the brand. Never. The brand is clear from beginning to end of each ad. In this version, the alliteration of Jake and Drake from State Farm is simply brilliant, as is the way they utter, multiple times, the iconic tag line "Like a Good Neighbor, State Farm is there" at the end.

Although I absolutely love the Jason Alexander hoodie ad[15], it is a failure from a brand recall perspective to me. While it makes me stop, watch, guffaw and smile every time it comes on, I still cannot remember the brand. Must be for a laundry detergent, correct? Yep, it's Tide. But I didn't recall that until I looked up the YouTube link just now to share with you.

So, I'm curious, what were your favorite ads and why?

Have a terrific weekend and thanks for all you do,
Amy

◯ REFLECTION

That State Farm commercial still is one of my favorites and most memorable. In fact, this email sparked a new interview question. I close out every screening interview with the final question, "What is your favorite ad and why?" I get the most interesting answers and it helps me understand the candidate's personality and interests, as well as their idea of what makes a good ad. It's far more insightful than telling me your greatest strengths and weaknesses.

✉ Subject: Happiness

Date: Friday, February 26, 2021, 6:09 p.m.

Team,

I am smiling at the end of this week. What an incredible week. So much excitement and so much progress. I can feel the momentum. And hope you can too. This week's ICC theme was "Happiness," with a few quotes to reflect on:

- *"Happiness is not something ready-made. It comes from your own actions."* —Dalai Lama XIV
- *"Talk about your blessings more than you talk about your problems."* —Anonymous
- *"True happiness is. . . to enjoy the present, without anxious dependence upon the future."* —Lucius Annaeus Seneca

Indeed, there is much to be happy about this week.

From crossing the 65,000-vaccinations mark today to the spectacular grand opening of the Emory Orthopaedics and Spine Center at Flowery Branch with the Atlanta Falcons yesterday. From reviewing and deciding upon radio together and locking in production and script approval for our new TV ad. Even the glimpses of spring with the days of sunshine and near 70-degree weather.

Each offers a chance to celebrate and enjoy the present.

For me though, the highlight of the week was hearing the joy in your voices at Staff meeting on Monday, sharing your gratitude for each other and celebrating the incredible team we've become. It made me beam from ear to ear then and still has me smiling now.

I am so proud of all you have accomplished and am so energized for the road ahead.

Thank you for all you do,
Amy

◯ REFLECTION

Emory Healthcare is the official team health care provider for the Atlanta Falcons. We built a care facility on the grounds of their Flowery Branch training facility, very similar to the Emory Sports Medicine Complex with the Atlanta Hawks. Construction continued throughout the pandemic. It seems construction stops for nothing. And we held our grand opening outside. It was the first time I saw some of my colleagues in person since the pandemic began.

Also, in 2018 when Emory Healthcare acquired DeKalb Medical, I had a newly expanded team. The teams had a very hard time jelling and working together. Part of that was due to our being in different locations and part due to the fact that for our first year, we operated marketing separately.

We didn't have a fully integrated team until September and October 2019. So, I adopted a practice I heard one of our palliative care physicians use with her team: starting every staff meeting going around the room and having each person share a moment of gratitude, either professionally or personally. It is a wonderful experience worth the time it takes. This remains an important part of our monthly staff meetings.

✉ Subject: Pandemic Silver Linings

Date: Friday, March 12, 2021, 5:09 p.m.

Team,

For many, yesterday marked the 12-month anniversary of the coronavirus pandemic in the United States. For me, two additional dates stand out: March 13 and March 17.

- March 11 is the day the WHO declared COVID-19 a global pandemic.

- March 13 is the day travel bans went into place and we were all worried if Mark and Becky would make it back into the States from Vietnam. It's also the day we decided to suspend elective surgeries and outpatient appointments.

- March 17 was the last time I sat in the fourth-floor conference room at Decatur Plaza. (After everyone went remote on the 16th, our marketing leaders had one last in-office day to coordinate our new remote environment.)

Much can be said for all of the challenges encountered in the last 12 months. And most certainly we need to pause, reflect and remember the lives lost, directly or indirectly, to COVID-19 throughout our state, nation and the world.

However, I want to spend today celebrating and reflecting on the good things that emerged from the pandemic. I like to call these "pandemic silver linings."

Every Storm Runs Out of Rain

I was on a call earlier this week where we were each asked to share one positive thing to come out of the pandemic. These silver linings included:

- *More time spent with kids*
- *Gaining 10 hours a week back from commute time*
- *Wearing jeans everyday*
- *Rest from the hustle and bustle of frequent work travel*
- *Having time to tend to home and garden*

For me? I shared our team's transformation from a group of individual contributors to the incredible high performing team we are now. To quote Dane from earlier today, "We can accomplish anything when we stick together as a team." Yes, indeed. You are a testament to that.

So, I'd love to hear your positive things, whether personal or professional. *What is your pandemic silver lining?*

Enjoy the beautiful weekend ahead of us,
Amy

✉@ **Subject: Hope Springs Eternal**

Date: Friday, March 19, 2021, 6:18 p.m.

Team,

Today marks the last day of winter. And, in less than 12 hours, at precisely 5:37 a.m. tomorrow, the vernal equinox will occur, welcoming a much-awaited first day of spring.

I realize this happens every year, but somehow the dawning of Spring 2021 feels. . .well. . .so much more.

Last year, we were barely a week into quarantine, with a heck of a lot of uncertainty ahead of us, when winter flipped to spring on March 19. No one truly knew what lied ahead. It was hard to feel hopeful with so much unknown, so much fear and so much anxiety.

A full 12 months later and everything feels different. Just like Mother Nature is carefully stretching her arms from a long winter's nap—tiny sprouts emerging from the ground, buds beginning to bloom—so are we carefully finding our way out of the pandemic.

Hope, although not ever truly gone, has fully arrived. And that light at the end of the tunnel shines more brightly each and every day.

Thanks to science, care, determination, and the drive of the human spirit, we are witnessing tremendous progress against COVID-19.

Georgia's positivity rate has dropped to 5% and our infection rate is well below 1.00. Even better, vaccine supply is constant and growing, with 23% of U.S. population receiving at least one dose. At our nation's current rate of vaccination, 75% of our population (the amount needed for herd immunity) will be achieved in five months.

While we still have a ways to go to be completely out of the pandemic, today I can confidently say hope springs eternal. As always, thank you for the role each of you play in improving lives and providing hope.

Happy Spring,
Amy

 REFLECTION

According to the journal *Nature*[16], we never did achieve herd immunity, and it is unlikely that we ever will.

📩 **Subject: Another Spring**

Date: Friday, March 26, 2021, 5:36 p.m.

Team,

Wednesday, we had our bimonthly senior leader meeting. Topics ranged from DEI to Constructive Culture to Epic to Finances and our Balanced Scorecard. A healthy mix of right-brained and left-brained topics. As it should—all great organizations need both to thrive.

During the culture topic, one leader spoke on resiliency, sharing theory, resources, and reminding us of the importance of focusing on our own resiliency to fight back against burnout.

He also gave us homework, challenging the 500 of us on the call to spend four minutes connecting with the arts. Specifically, he asked us all to find time to listen, purposefully, to Nina Simone's "Another Spring."

I did so this morning—holy cow is this song packed! The lyrics. The abstract piano intro. Her breathy speech going into lyrical singing. The joy and the heartache. The slight modulation to another brighter key as she sings about "Another Spring." There is a lot here.

For me, I didn't think one song could capture the feeling of the past 12 months. But "Another Spring" captured in music what I was trying to accomplish in words last week.

I'm thankful each and every one of us is here to experience another spring. I was reminded yesterday how quickly another spring can be stolen—learning during a meeting of the death of a young employee who lost her battle against COVID in February.

So, let's do everything we can to help each other, our patients, and our families ensure that we all can enjoy *another spring* this year, and for many more to come.

Thank you for all you do,
Amy

 REFLECTION

"Another Spring" is magnificent. I love Ella and Nat and Etta, and I thought I knew Nina Simone. But clearly, I did not. This was pure performance art. I remember lying on my yoga mat in my guest room office, listening to this through my earbuds, eyes closed. Pure magic. Honestly, I cannot describe it. Just pop in your earbuds, close your eyes, lay back and experience Nina—The High Priestess of Soul.

✉ **Subject: If you want a rainbow. . .**

Date: Friday, April 16, 2021, 5:51 p.m.

Team,

What a difference a year makes.

Do you remember Spring Break 2020? Me neither. It was the spring break that never happened. We were only three weeks into our pandemic journey and shelter-in-place canceled nearly everybody's plans.

Though still not entirely out of the pandemic, we are finally clearly on the other side. The promise and science of vaccines held true, and, due to YOUR work, Emory Healthcare has delivered more than 135,000 COVID-19 vaccinations to date. That means more lives saved, more families and friends reunited.

Did you know some have dubbed their first post-vaccine vacation a "Vacci-moon"?

We spent ours finally making it to Dollywood, albeit a year later than planned. Some of you may recall I wrote about my newfound fascination with Dolly Parton in a "Decompressing with Dolly" Friday message last May. Listening to *Dolly Parton's America* during walks around the neighborhood was my much needed escape during shelter-in-place.

That, plus her $1 million donation to support COVID efforts at Vanderbilt that led to the development of the Moderna vaccine, made the delayed trip to Dollywood so much more meaningful.

I came across this quote of hers on our last day and thought it captured the year and the moment perfectly—*"The way I see it, if you want the rainbow, you gotta put up with the rain."*

We're not out of the woods yet, with many more vaccinations needed to get to herd immunity, but perhaps this pandemic storm has nearly run out of its rain too. I see many rainbows ahead.

Thank you for all you do,
Amy

💬 REFLECTION

Fully vaccinated, I stood as a literal physical barrier in roller coaster lines shielding my half-vaxxed husband and unvaxxed 15-year old. Pediatric vaccines weren't available yet. We wore masks outside in the park. There were six-foot markers that no one paid attention to and hand sanitizer stations everywhere (though often empty).

Dollywood staff stopped to sanitize the rides after a certain amount of runs.

At the hotel, we decidedly did not eat in any restaurants, getting all of our food to go and we were horrified by how many people hung out by and got into the pool!

That said, Dollywood is AWESOME. The roller coasters fabulous. I'm ready to go back.

✉@ **Subject: Justice**

Date: Friday, April 23, 2021, 6:52 p.m.

Team,

I've been thinking a lot this week about what to write for this Friday send-off.

Early in the week I was ready to focus on justice and the step forward we made in fighting racial injustice with the jury's powerful decision in the Chauvin trial. But news of the deaths of Ma'Khia Bryant, Daunte Wright and Adam Toledo, combined with the March mass shooting that targeted our own Asian-American community, remind us just how many more steps we have to go.

So, how do we reconcile this? I don't think you can reconcile it, but rather we can learn from it. We can focus on how we as individuals respond to and think about racial injustice. As well as the role our institution plays in making diversity, equity and inclusion a focal point for our own employees, and especially for our patients and their families.

I also looked to our team. I am incredibly proud of the diversity of our team. From BIPOC to LGBTQ, along with religious, gender, and generational diversity, our small but mighty team reflects the richness of the American spirit I know and love. Each and every day we learn from each other, building upon our differences to make our team and ourselves stronger for it.

And in doing so we can reflect that richness of diversity to our patients and families through our messaging, creative, and marketing strategy. Helping those that know Emory Healthcare and those that don't know us yet, truly understand our core drive to improve lives and provide hope for the health of our entire community, right here in our home city of Atlanta and home state of Georgia.

So, as you enter this weekend, give thanks for the progress made this week, give a moment of pause for the lives lost and focus on the hope in your hearts to continue improving lives—yours, ours, and our community's.

Thank you for all you do. I am proud to serve alongside each and every one of you.

Amy

Subject: A Splendid Gift

Date: Friday, May 7, 2021, 6:16 p.m.

Team,

Yesterday, May 6, marked National Nurses Day, and kicked off a week of celebrating nurses worldwide. As I took to the Internet to find an interesting tidbit or story to share, I came across this quote from Florence Nightingale:

"Live life when you have it. Life is a splendid gift—there is nothing small about it."

I found it so apropos to both the lessons of the past 12 months and reflecting on Mother's Day.

A year of living among COVID-19 has reminded us how quickly life, and living, can change. Yet, the circle of life extends far beyond the impact of coronavirus, with lives entering and leaving our world every day—for thousands of years before and thousands of years to come. Which is what brings me to Mother's Day.

Our mothers gave us a splendid gift—life. The best way we can honor them is to live our lives to the fullest.

Happy Mother's Day,
Amy

✉@ **Subject: The Real MVP**

Date: Friday, May 14, 2021, 5:44 p.m.

Team,

A year ago on May 15, 2020, I took this picture to celebrate #nationalhealthcareweek and honor the amazing team we have.

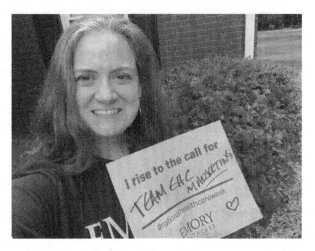

You all rose to the call then—and have continued to rise to the call every single day of this shared pandemic journey.

Our only certainty this time last year? *The only way out is through.*

How glorious does it feel to know we are nearly through?

- Vaccines are in full supply
- The CDC says fully vaccinated individuals no longer need to mask (except in specific situations), which meant a great Team Marketing reunion for many of you yesterday.
- And Emory's COVID-19 survival rate is among the best in the nation!

The head of our ICU and Critical Care units shared the news this week.

Comparing mortality rates (the lower the number the better): Emory Healthcare's average as a system is .66 (and as low as .57 at Emory University Hospital). The national hospital mortality rate average is .82 and .85 among academic medical centers.

Think of how many individual lives are part of that nearly .20 Emory difference. So many lives saved, and families reunited thanks to the incredible teams at Emory Healthcare.

YOU are integral to that success. People chose Emory because of **your** work. People are getting vaccinated because of **your** work. People choose Emory for their health care needs, because of **your** work.

So, a year older and six inches grayer, and prouder than ever of you, I restaged last year's health care week selfie.

Emory Healthcare Marketing truly is the REAL MVP in my book.

Happy Health Care Week,
Amy

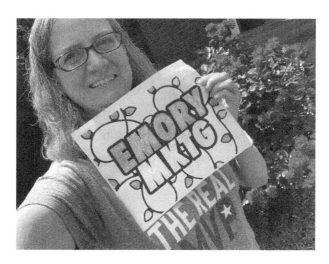

✉️ **Subject: Reflecting on Memorial Day**

Date: Friday, May 28, 2021, 4:32 p.m.

Team,

Every Memorial Day, I think of my maternal grandfather, Daniel Reisch. He was a Chief Master Sergeant in the U.S. Air Force and I never got to meet him.

He died of a heart attack at the young age of 56, the year before I was born.

I know him only through the stories my mom and dad (who were high school sweethearts) and my late grandmother would share with me and my sisters. I have always been fascinated by my grandfather. I'm sure I share some of his traits and understand my mother inherited her calmness, sharp intellect and love of reading from him.

Six years after Daniel Reisch died, the "first balloon angioplasty on a coronary artery was performed by Andreas Gruentzig in Zurich, Switzerland."

Dr. Gruentzig eventually immigrated to the United States and became faculty at Emory's School of Medicine. Recruited in the 1980s by physicians many of us know and have worked with: Dr. Doug Morris, Dr. Spencer King and Dr. John Douglas, Jr. Together this quartet of pioneers built Emory's internationally renowned heart and vascular program.

I often wonder if I would have had the chance to meet my grandfather had these important advances in medicine come a decade earlier. Today angioplasty is a common routine procedure that saves millions of lives, with more than 850,000 performed annually in the United States.

Despite these advances, heart disease is still the number one killer of Americans, with more than 650,000 losing their lives to heart disease in 2019. That's more in one year, than the 593,000 American lives lost to COVID-19.

Which is why the work our team is doing to drive heart and vascular volumes is so important. While the pressure to drive volumes is real, understand that pressure is driven by our core purpose to improve lives and provide hope.

The work you are doing to identify Georgians at risk makes a difference. The creative messaging is equally as important to drive conversion. The 1% response rate we expect equals lives impacted—lives saved—in their decision to take action and take that action at Emory.

Thank you for your continued dedication to our patient-and family-centered care mission. Your work is saving this generation of Daniel Reisches and I know their granddaughters will thank you for it.

Thank you for all you do,
Amy

✉ **Subject: To Fellowship**

Date: Friday, June 4, 2021, 5:49 p.m.

Team,

How wonderful it was to see so many of you in *real life* yesterday at Brick Store Pub!

While I had seen a few of you in person at various events over the past year, this was the first time I had seen many of you in more than 15 months. It warmed my heart to have us all gathered around the tables together, enjoying each other, laughing, telling stories, and wishing our dear colleagues, Melissa and Shannon, well on their newest adventures.

For those of you who were not able to join us, Shannon cooked up a few surprise guests as well.

Sitting at the end of the table when I arrived was the one and only Michelle (my former admin). She and her husband are doing well enjoying a new camper they bought and checking out camp sites across the state. Stefanie also joined us, and I was glad to be able to wish her well in person, as I missed out on the last gathering. And, some of you may also remember Jamarcus, who walked in surprising us all. He interned with us in 2018, quickly becoming an extended member of our Marketing family.

Alas, I did not snap any pics or selfies, so I don't have any proof, but it was a wonderful time. The Virtual Happy Hours are fun, but nothing holds a candle to the camaraderie of being together in person. I'm thankful for the vaccines and the scientists at Emory

Healthcare and academic medical centers across the country that made safe celebrating possible.

To Melissa, Shannon, and Stefanie—we already miss you, but we are also incredibly proud of you. It's truly my pleasure to see you thrive and grow in your careers.

Thank you for all you have done for Emory. You are forever part of the EHC Marketing family.

Thank you for all you do,
Amy

✉@ **Subject: A June for Reflection**

Date: Friday, June 18, 2021, 5:42 p.m.

Team,

June gives us much to reflect on with Pride month, Juneteenth, and Father's Day upon us.

I am embarrassed to admit that I only became familiar with Juneteenth last year. I'm shocked it wasn't part of my education when we learned about the Emancipation Proclamation and the end of slavery. In today's age of instant messaging and social media, it is hard to comprehend that message of freedom took two and a half years to reach Texas. I still cannot wrap my mind around it.

Emory itself has our own history to reckon with. I respect the University and School of Medicine's acknowledgement of this and apology to Dr. Marion G. Hood yesterday. For those of you not familiar, he was denied application to our School of Medicine based on his skin color that year.

I also had the immense fortune to meet and learn from Verdelle Bellamy, during my stint as communications director for Emory's Nell Hodgson Woodruff School of Nursing. Ms. Bellamy was one of the first two African American students to graduate from Emory, earning her master's degree in nursing in 1963. Sadly, she died in 2015, but leaves a lasting legacy at Emory and the nursing profession.

I still have much to learn about racial, gender and religious diversity, equity and inclusion. As a white woman, I will never truly experience the world from the lens of others who don't look like me. But I can promise that I will continue to learn, never stop seeking to understand, and commit to being an ally.

I find the convergence of Pride, Juneteenth, and Father's Day in one month poetic. After all, a parent's greatest hope is a better world for their children. I am thankful for the progress we are making and hope that momentum continues for generations to come.

Happy Pride, Happy Juneteenth and Happy Father's Day,
Amy

✉️ **Subject: Freedom**

Date: Friday, July 2, 2021, 4:15 p.m.

Team,

As we enter the weekend looking forward to celebrating our nation's Independence Day, I cannot help but think how profound the timing of our final COVID-19 ICC is.

The focused work we have done as a system to battle COVID-19 over the past 16 months has come to an end. While the virus is still out there, and likely will be for some time, we can finally close the pandemic chapter we have been living.

Monday's ICC was an emotional one as we all marveled at how far we've come, as individuals, as a system, and most importantly as a team. While we fought a formidable opponent, we also made ourselves stronger. And we saved more than 12,000 lives. In fact, we learned Monday, that Emory Healthcare's critical care survival rate is quite literally the best in the world when it comes to COVID-19.

Dr. B graciously, deliberately, and at times emotionally thanked each work group for their contributions in the fight against COVID-19. About YOU, he said: "Thank you for the incredible work your team created. Powerful and important messaging our communities and patients needed at each stage of the journey."

Do you remember this time last year? Shelter-in-place had come and gone. Yet we were still quarantining at home and about to face an enormous spike in COVID-19 cases, with no end in sight. Our financial state was dire with several of us taking furloughs.

We mourned our Emory colleagues who fell victim to the virus. The promise of vaccines still a wild fantasy.

How incredible to look back and see how far we have come. Since December more than 2.9 billion doses of COVID-19 vaccines have been delivered. Nearly 3 billion!

With the vaccines comes freedom. And now, our country can enjoy a rebirth of sorts this weekend.

Thank you for everything you have done to make this freedom a reality for our patients, our community, and ourselves. It's time to celebrate.

Happy Independence Day,
Amy

REFLECTION

I remember this day well. We thought we were finally done with the pandemic. We ended our incident command center, intent on getting back to business as usual. It certainly was a time to celebrate. But as we know all too well now, it was not the end.

We haven't even gotten to the variants yet!

✉ Subject: Always Be You

Date: Friday, July 9, 2021, 4:41 p.m.

Team,

For the past 16 months, we've been a lot of things to a lot of people. COVID-19 changed how we worked, how we lived, how we played, even who we are.

As we enter a new post-pandemic, or endemic, phase, we will go through another transition. For some it will be easy to make the shift to yet another new normal, while others will find it harder to let go, still needing to grieve or process what happened to our world.

No matter where you are in that spectrum, remember one thing: Always be you. Allow yourself to grieve COVID-19 if that's what you need. Allow yourself to celebrate and jump for joy if that's what you need. Only you know what you need, and you should always listen to your heart, and take care of yourself.

For me, I am nearly giddy with excitement to see my family this weekend. While I've been able to see my parents, I have not seen my two sisters nor their families in two years, almost to the date. My youngest nephew was two and a half the last time I hugged him; he'll be five in August. I'm thankful my family, so far, escaped the grips of COVID-19; but I recognize how lucky we are and that there are many families out there whose summer reunions will be bittersweet with family members missing from their tables, whether it be due to COVID-19 or other reasons.

And so, I find myself somewhere in between grief and joy. But in 2021 I am focusing hard on being myself, taking care of myself, laughing, loving, creating, and letting go. Have a wonderful weekend and week ahead. See you on the 20th.

Thank you for being you,
Amy

 PRO TIP

The word "endemic" means regularly occurring in an area, which is truly where we are now with COVID-19 in our world.

✉ Subject: Grit & Grace

Date: Friday, July 30, 2021, 5:31 p.m.

Admittedly, I am going to plagiarize a bit this week. But this passage from Gary Burnison's weekly email really captures my thinking lately.

Where grit meets grace. When the going gets tough, and the way forward is shrouded in uncertainty, grit can push us through. It's the tenacious drive that makes us resilient against all odds. But grit, alone, cannot do the job—especially when leading others.

Grit reports to grace—the real sovereign. In the face of failure, grace assures us that we will not only be OK, but also actually get better. And, amid success, grace guards us against self-importance. No matter what happens the only question is: **Do we have the grit to be graceful?**

For those of you unfamiliar, Gary Burnison is CEO of Korn Ferry, a global organizational consulting firm, and author of several leadership books. Many of us receive his weekly blog in our inboxes on Monday mornings. Cheryl has been kind to say she enjoys bookending her work week with emails from me and Gary. (Cheryl—sorry this is a repeat for you!)

Leadership is a never-ending journey. And like life, it has its highs, lows, and unexpected twists and turns.

All of us are leaders, even if we do not serve in a traditional leadership role. We are peer leaders, sports leaders, community leaders, family leaders, even leaders among friends. Each of us knows the grit involved and Gary so importantly reminds us of grace.

No one more embodied grit and grace this week than Simone Biles.

I eagerly stayed up late over the weekend to watch her live qualifiers. Excited to see the GOAT in action again. Like the world, I worried when she stumbled on a few routines. I thought nothing of it, however, and expected she'd rebound in team competition. So, I was stunned when Fred shared during Huddle that she had withdrawn.

I have spent the days since consuming content about her—the twisties, social support from athletes—and been awed by her EQ and leadership. She indeed has the grit to be graceful.

May we all be inspired by Simone to keep grace front and center in our own leadership.

Thank you for all you do,
Amy

✉ Subject: Bending with the Wind

Date: Friday, August 6, 2021, 4:56 p.m.

Team,

Earlier this week I heard a great quote from Bruce Lee.

"Notice that the stiffest tree is most easily cracked, while the bamboo or willow survives by bending with the wind."

People often ask me the key to success working at Emory Healthcare. Resourcefulness always ranks at the top of my list. But adaptability is a close second.

Health care and marketing are industries that never stand still. What is new today is old tomorrow.

Whether it is new scientific discoveries changing protocols or emerging digital trends changing consumer behavior, things are constantly evolving.

The current surging of the Delta variant and changing CDC mask guidance for vaccinated individuals are evidence of this in motion. As are the changing habits of how the world is consuming Olympic Games coverage.

Not too long-ago families gathered around the TV to catch primetime coverage of the Games as a scheduled event. No one cared if coverage wasn't live because we didn't know the results. Today, we can stream the Olympics 24/7, watch live on multiple TV channels and get immediate push notifications from numerous apps, web sites, or social media channels.

Indeed, what was new yesterday is old today.

We must emulate the willow to find balance in the midst of this constant flow of change. Our strong roots always anchoring us, but our branches and leaves flow so we can continue to adapt and thrive in the world around us.

Thank you for all you do,
Amy

REFLECTION

Remember the 2020 Olympics and the UEFA EUROS were postponed to 2021 due to the pandemic. It is eerie and amazing to be editing this book with both going full-steam ahead in 2024!

✉@ **Subject: Inch by Inch**

Date: Friday, August 20, 2021, 4:08 p.m.

Team,

Are you tired? I am.

This fourth surge is a real bummer.

And in ways it feels worse than the first three. The first we had adrenaline, focus, and worldwide unity on the crisis at hand.

It was cute we thought it would be over in eight weeks. Here we are 18 months and four surges later—it's exhausting.

I don't like being taken for granted. I'm sure you don't either. But isn't that what it feels like now?

People have moved on. The pandemic is (was) over. Time to get back to normal.

Yet here we are. Gone are the cheers. Gone is the unity. Gone the focus on a common foe.

We held up our end of the bargain, but not all of society did. And now our health systems are overburdened once again. Our COVID beds filled with unvaccinated people.

My heart breaks for those who are infected and didn't have access to vaccines and wanted them. That is why our journey continues.

My heart and head hurt at how to help those on the fence take the leap of science and get vaccinated. Also, part of our journey.

Yet we will take care of them all. Doing all we can to save their lives. And when we cannot, ensure that no one dies alone on our watch. It's our calling. It's what we do—improving lives and providing hope.

There are days I can manage this dissonance. And others when I cannot. But Wednesday, during an online workout (pandemic silver lining!), the trainer shared this quote: *"Yard by yard, life is hard. Inch by inch, life's a cinch."*

I needed that. Change doesn't happen in big fell swoops. It happens little by little, bit by bit. It is the constant chipping away that creates major progress.

Bit by bit our community vaccination efforts in underserved communities have saved more than 5,600 lives. Thirty-some this week in Toco Hills alone. In total that's more people than those occupying our current COVID beds.

And, think of the innumerable small bits of progress our team has made over the past three years since DeKalb joined Emory Healthcare.

Think back to this time in 2018. . .We were a newly formed team, finding our way and managing together the Decatur Book Festival and three signage unveilings in a single day.

Last night, we presented—**as a team**—one of the most sophisticated marketing plans and presentations to our leadership team that I can remember.

We did that. YOU did that. Bit by Bit. One step at a time.

When you simply focus on one step at a time, you look back and realize just how far you've come.

I'm proud of you. Of all of you, for the work you've done to build our marketing program to what it is today, and for everything you continue to do to fight the virus.

I may still be tired, but I am also proud, beaming and inspired.

Thank you for all you do,
Amy

✉ Subject: Imagination, Hope and Courage

Date: Friday, August 27, 2021, 4:51 p.m.

Team,

Last Friday I started my day at Winship to interview a candidate for their lead marketing and communications position.

I have come to love my "WFW" (Work from Work) days. As much as I love working from home, nothing beats experiencing our brand in-person. Our staff and providers never cease to amaze me in their commitment to patient-and family-centered care. Everyone I encountered was compassionately engaged with our patients and their visitors, and warmly greeted me as well.

That morning I decided to take the four flights of stairs to Winship's administrative suite, instead of the elevator. Even though I have walked these stairs countless times in my 16+ years with Emory, the core values embedded in them never cease to inspire. Even more so during the pandemic.

This was my first trek up and down them since we left for quarantine in March 2020.

Translation, Imagination, Hope, Courage—constant words of inspiration for our cancer patients, their families and the staff, researchers, and providers who work in that building.

Yet these words and values transcend. Ever more so meaningful as we navigate a world with COVID-19.

With each surge, our **courage** tested. With each new scientific discovery, our **translation** needed. Our **imagination** used daily to increase vaccination rates or urge people to seek care at Emory. And, always, we **hope** for a better tomorrow.

You each embody these values in our daily work as a marketing team, and in our organization's never-ending quest to improve lives and provide hope.

Thank you for all you do and enjoy your weekend,
Amy

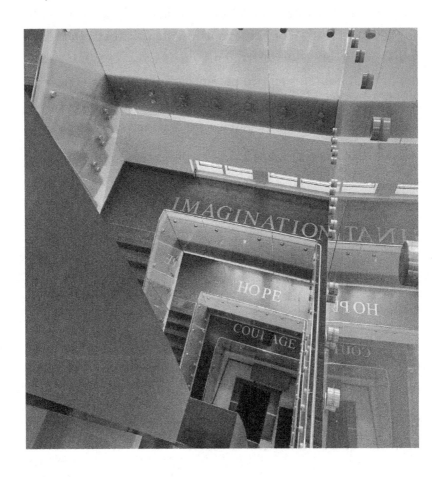

✉ Subject: Happy New Year!

Date: Friday, September 3, 2021, 11:55 am

Team,

No one can top DJ Jazzy Jared's ringing in the new fiscal year during Wednesday's huddle. I'm still dancing to the "Happy" earworm! (P.S. Do you remember Arby's 15 minutes of social media fame related to Pharrell's hat?)

However, I personally wanted to take a moment to reflect on a truly remarkable year. Our first full fiscal year, in fact, in the midst of a global pandemic.

A couple weeks ago I wrote about making progress bit by bit. When I look back on FY21, our many bits accomplished some pretty big things.

Here are just a few of the things we've accomplished as a team:

- Captured and engaged more than 213,000 leads
- Sent more than 11 million emails
- Sent more than 75,000 pieces of direct mail using 12 propensity models
- Ran three broadcast campaigns: Feel Safe, Get It Done, Olympics
- Smoked our HealthSource goal of a 30% increase, achieving a 130% increase overall
- Generated more than $22 million in marketing-influenced contribution margin

- Produced more than 900 pieces of content

- Completed nearly 2,000 jobs –> 1,922 exactly

- Performed 16,152 tasks to complete those jobs

- Won many awards, including Best in Show for our "Rise to the Call" campaign

- Converted and acquired 2,783 new patients, which represents $1.2 billion (yes, billion) in customer lifetime value, should they stay loyal to Emory, not to mention improved and better health outcomes by their choosing Emory

- Led 11 community vaccine events inoculating 1,100 who might not have otherwise had access to the vaccine

- Helped Emory Healthcare deliver more than 180,000 vaccinations to our patients, the general public and our staff

- Welcomed three new members to Team EHC Marketing

- Welcomed new babies, grandbabies and furry friends to our extended Marketing family

As you enjoy a well-deserved, and hopefully restful, long Labor Day weekend, take a minute to toast your accomplishments and take pride in knowing your work has most certainly improved lives and provided hope.

Thank you for all you do,
Amy

✉ Subject: An anniversary we never wanted

Date: Friday, September 10, 2021, 4:44 p.m.

Twenty years ago tonight I sat on the stage of the Atlanta Civic Center looking out into an empty audience.

Chairs lined the stage apron facing the curtain, as the Atlanta Opera's leadership spoke optimistically of a new era for the company—moving from the historic Fox Theatre to be the premiere resident of the Boisfeuillet Jones Atlanta Civic Center.

We purposely held our board meeting on the stage to signal the significance and excitement of the moment. We dropped our season ticket renewals for the 2002 Season the same day—September 10, 2001.

We left the board meeting excited for this new growth phase for the Opera. Little did we know 12 hours later our world and lives would change forever.

Everyone remembers where they were on September 11, 2001.

I woke up normally—driving from my Peachtree Hills condo to our Opera Center in Midtown and listening to The Morning X (remember 99X?). A worrisome news break about a plane crashing into the World Trade Center came on as I fought rush hour traffic down Spring Street.

Something didn't feel right. By the time I got to work a second plane hit. My heart sank. I knew immediately something terrible was happening.

I parked my car and went straight to our conference room. There I joined our costume designer and others gathered around the fuzzy TV news feed to take in what was happening.

All of us know what happened from there. Our world changed. Dramatically.

I think a LOT about that day. For me, it became a life- and career-defining moment. But for far too many, it brought heartbreak. Needless lives lost, families forever changed, cityscapes demolished and many now still suffering from illness whether it be cancer, respiratory disease, PTSD, or other mental health challenges.

Each year I make a point to honor those lives lost and impacted by September 11, often taking a moment of silence during Huddle.

Tomorrow when I reflect on the American lives lost from and impacted by 9/11, I also will mourn the freedom lost by Afghan women. For the past 20 years, they've experienced freedom and opportunity, only to find themselves oppressed again, after the Taliban has retaken power and repealed two decades of freedom from repression. Fearing for their lives. I pray for their peace, safety and equality.

I wish there was a way I could help improve their lives and provide hope. Instead I will channel my energy where I know I can make an impact—focusing on the work we are doing to improve the health of individuals and communities here in Georgia.

Yesterday Dr. B. shared a Jewish teaching *"that someone who saves a life saves the world."* I am holding that message close on this

20th anniversary of September 11. Knowing each life we save by encouraging vaccination or helping people choose Emory Healthcare is indeed saving the world.

Thank you,
Amy

P.S. We all have our September 11 memories, haunts and stories— if you have one you'd like to share, I'd be honored to hear it.

✉ Subject: A Day of Atonement

Date: Friday, September 17, 2021, 5:43 p.m.

Our Jewish friends, patients and colleagues observed Yom Kippur this week. While I have known of this holiday for many years, I took the time last night to learn a little more.

I often confuse the differences between Rosh Hashanah and Yom Kippur. I know one is a new year, but can never remember which one.

For those of you in the same boat—Rosh Hashanah honors the new year. Yom Kippur is the most holy Jewish day of the year, a day of atonement. Both are connected.

From the jewishunpacked.com[17] blog—"Gmar chatima tova" means "a good final sealing" in Hebrew. Typically said between the two holidays, it "is based on the belief that our fates are 'written' on Rosh Hashanah and 'sealed' on Yom Kippur. This expresses the wish that someone will be inscribed in the Book of Life."

Turning more specifically to Yom Kippur[18], Chabad.org shares that "Beyond specific actions, Yom Kippur is dedicated to introspection, prayer, and asking God for forgiveness."

I find this dedication beautiful and pure. As an introvert (I'm sure some of you may be surprised to hear me say this), a day fully dedicated to introspection sounds breathtaking. A day to remember why we are all on this Earth and to reflect on our own purpose, our own actions, and practice forgiveness.

Forgiving ourselves for any shortcomings we see. Finding confidence from our strengths. Humbled in acknowledging our weaknesses. Forgiving others for their actions, intentional or not.

After 18 months of pandemic living and seeing how the virus has divided our country, the arrival of Yom Kippur this year couldn't be more poignant.

Whether we are Jewish or not, our collective global society could use a day of atonement. A day to pause, to reflect, to be introspective, see the other side, and forgive. Beginning a new year on a fresh page.

For it is in our similarities that we thrive, through our differences we learn and grow, and in forgiveness that we find peace.

A belated G'mar Tov all of you,
Amy

✉ **Subject: Experiencing Emory Healthcare**

Date: Friday, October 1, 2021, 6:22 p.m.

Team,

Monday I mentioned being alternately grateful for my WFW and WFH days, enjoying the flexibility and benefits of our hybrid model.

Yesterday Miranda and I had a powerful WFW day, where we experienced firsthand the work our care teams do every day to improve lives and provide hope.

Since Miranda needed to pick up her ID badge from the Midtown security office, I asked our Midtown hospital's CEO, if he'd be willing to give us a behind-the-scenes tour of the hospital. He was gracious to oblige and spent nearly an hour of his day showing us around.

We started with a tour of the fourth floor cardiac unit, continued past the two aviaries and saw the incredible transformation of the old Linden lot into the new Winship tower. From there we walked past the Davis-Fischer building to take in the grandeur of the new "Garage-Mahal," past the ED and back to the Orr Building. A landmark building, the W. W. Orr Building, is also our Marketing Team's former home and where I started my EHC career.

The very highlight of our tour was our visit to the NICU.

We were not expecting to see patient care so up close and personal, but I am forever grateful for the experience. We walked past many intricate beds with tiny babies fighting for their lives. Each as precious as you can imagine.

Along the way, we encountered a physician from Children's Healthcare of Atlanta (CHOA), who took the time to explain the magic that happens there.

Emory University Hospital Midtown, CHOA and Grady are the only hospitals in the entire state of Georgia that are part of the Angel II Neonatal Transport. We are the only hospitals equipped to deal with the most complex newborns, whether prematurely born (some are as tiny as a single pound!) or dealing with asphyxiation from challenging deliveries.

There are special ambulances from this network that bring these babies in need to our facilities from all over the state of Georgia. Their specially designed transport beds costing $400,000 each and each of the 48 intricate beds in our Midtown NICU costing $125,000. Not to mention the countless dedicated staff on the hospital and transport teams that care for these precious babies.

Sadly, not all of these babies make it through, despite the incredible care. Tough but compassionate conversations are had with the parents to help them make decisions they never imagined they'd have to make.

I say this not to depress, but rather to inspire. A reminder of the incredible honor and privilege we have that this type of care is the product we market. Not butter, not hotels, not sandwiches, not cars, but **CARE**. Compassionate, ethical, innovative and market-leading health care.

So when you are having a hard day or feeling disconnected from your work, put on your badge and go sit in a waiting room or walk around one of our facilities.

Take in everything around you. Help a lost patient or family member find where they are going, even if just to the closest information desk. See and feel the impact Emory Healthcare makes every day to improve lives and provide hope.

I bet you'll come to find you cherish your WFW days as well.

Thank you for all you do,
Amy

Subject: Dream Builders

Date: Friday, October 15, 2021, 5:45 p.m.

Team,

We all have hopes and dreams. Our early career selves see something that inspires. We dream of what seems to be an impossible dream.

And then, one day, you realize that dream wasn't so impossible after all.

In 1997, I moved to Atlanta—young, alone, driven, and naive. Excited to build my career in marketing and PR with The Atlanta Opera.

That year I attended my first AMA AMY Awards and sat mesmerized. Huge Atlanta-based national brands winning awards for incredible marketing campaigns. I wondered how on earth I could get the Opera among these ranks. I dreamed my own impossible dream that day to win an AMY.

(I mean, who doesn't want to win an award that is both their namesake and for the industry they love??)

But these awards don't come easily. Our Emory Healthcare team earned finalist honors for many years yet failed to cross the finish line in first place. Often losing to Piedmont Healthcare (grr...) or well-deserving, non-health care Atlanta brands.

So, this year, when we were nominated as finalists with nary a Piedmont finalist in sight, I thought, maybe, just maybe...this would be our year.

You know the story well by now. Cheryl and Denise represented our team at last week's awards ceremony and brought home our first AMY! Earning top honors for our "Rise to the Call" campaign. A fitting tribute in the wake of the pandemic. I'm told Denise gave an amazing Oscar-worthy speech accepting it.

As any good vacation will do, I completely forgot about the AMYs. So, as we were walking around the Magic Kingdom, I got a text message and photo of the award from Denise, saying: *"Boom. There you go."*

I am pretty sure I jumped for joy. And my boys will tell you I was grinning from Mickey-ear to Mickey-ear.

A 25-year-old girl dreamed an impossible dream, and nearly 30 years later, it came true. Even better to get the news in a magical place that promises dreams can come true. It really can happen to you!

Turns out it wasn't an impossible dream after all. Anything can be achieved with a great team, hard work, and perseverance. This team made it happen. *Your work and your effort brought this dream to life*. For that I am forever grateful.

It is fitting that the next day walking around Epcot, I encountered this message from Walt.

> *"The way to get started is to quit talking and begin doing."*
> — Walt Disney

This AMY Award belongs to all of us. **You are dream builders.**

And know that this is only the beginning—we are at the start of something BIG!

October 15, 2021, 5:45 p.m.

Thank you for all you do and never stop dreaming...
Amy

 PRO TIP

AMY is the abbreviation for Atlanta Marketer of the Year, given out by the American Marketing Association's Atlanta chapter.

REFLECTION

I attended my first AMA AMY Awards in the late 1990s after moving to Georgia for my position at The Atlanta Opera. I sat there in awe of these major brands, their campaigns and their work. Winning an AMY Award seemed far-fetched. But it became a personal goal: a marketer named Amy absolutely must win an AMY Award!

Fast forward to the late 2010s when I stepped into my leadership role with Emory Healthcare marketing. For several years, we earned Finalist creds, but never won. Always the bridesmaid, never the bride. So when Denise texted me our team finally won our first AMY, I really did jump for joy midstride at Disney. A year later, we won our second AMY.

This time I was in person with my team. I accepted the award on our team's behalf and shared the story with the crowd about my dream as a young marketer and Atlanta transplant coming true. Even better, it was due to the work we did with Matt Ryan and the Atlanta Falcons.

✉ Subject: Take me out to the ball game

Date: Friday, October 22, 2021, 5:58 p.m.

Team,

While I love soccer, baseball holds a special place in my sports heart.

My dad took me to my first baseball game at War Memorial Stadium in Buffalo shortly after we saw *The Natural*. Not everyone knows that movie was filmed in Buffalo. All of the baseball scenes shot in this stadium, then home to the Buffalo Bisons.

My dad eventually bought season tickets. We went to countless games there and followed the team to Pilot Field when they made their bid for an MLB expansion team. We lost our bid and I have hated the Colorado Rockies ever since...

My dad taught me everything I know about baseball. I remember learning to keep score from the stands. Learned the differences between the NL and AL, about the farm system, pitching signs, everything.

On every family vacation, my dad took me to a game at the local stadium, from the Grapefruit League to the Cactus League and many MLB games in between. I am so fortunate to have been to Fenway, Shea Stadium, and Comiskey Park. I got to see Reggie Jackson play at Exhibition Stadium in Toronto and Pete Rose play at Jack Murphy Stadium in San Diego. Memories of a lifetime.

I happily returned the favor nearly a decade ago, taking my dad to his first Atlanta Braves game at Turner Field. And when SunTrust Park opened, I gave him a hat for his birthday and told him we had a new stadium to see. Haven't been there yet together, but definitely on our father-daughter stadium bucket list.

I love to watch baseball. Nothing beats a live game, but watching the Braves on TV has become a staple in my self-care routine over the past five years. There's something calming about watching baseball that helps my mind relax and unwind. Perhaps it's the crack of the bat or the unmistakable sound of a home run ball coming off it.

The Braves are one win away from the World Series. One win! While they didn't close it out yesterday, here's hoping they can take care of business this weekend.

Go Braves!
Amy

REFLECTION

In 2022, cheering on the defending World Series champions, my father and I made it to SunTrust Park (now Truist Park) and crossed another stadium off the bucket list.

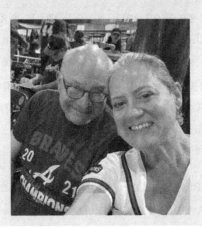

✉ Subject: Hello my beauties

Date: Friday, October 29, 2021, 5:25 p.m.

Hello My Beauties!

Maleficent here. I've absconded your leader so you will not be getting your standard Friday email from her.

I needed a human body to inhabit to compete among mere mortals in the Rockdale Magnet School for Science and Technology's annual Monster Dash 5K Run/Walk. Have to teach these kids a lesson in speed.

And I hear your leader is ditching you next week to "give a talk" in Las Vegas. A likely story. . .who really works in Vegas? Ahhhh, but if Sin City isn't one of Maleficent's favorite places!

Rest assured Amy will be back to her drab and dull Friday emails the following week. Until then, while the cat's away the mice can play!

—Maleficent

P.S. Alas, the 5K has been postponed due to threat of rain. I am not the Wicked Witch and rain does not hurt me. Cannot believe silly humans are afraid to run or walk in the mist. SMH. Perhaps I'll go for a stroll around the neighborhood and spook the neighbors instead!

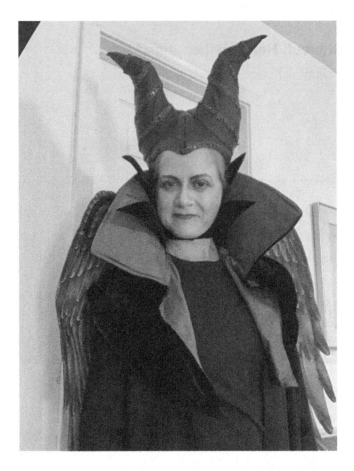

I did walk the neighborhood in my make-up, but not the wings or hat.

✉ Subject: With My Gratitude

Date: Friday, November 19, 2021, 4:07 p.m.

Team,

Well, it appears Maleficent really DID abscond with me. My Halloween 2021 is certainly one I'll never forget.

When the Emory Decatur Hospital ED team prepped me for surgery, including the lovely hair bonnet (sorry no pics exist. . .), I joked that I was going as a patient for Halloween.

In any case, I'm enormously thankful for the amazing care I received at Emory Decatur Hospital, and ever more thankful that DeKalb Medical became part of the Emory Healthcare family. Otherwise, I'd have ended up at Piedmont Rockdale and probably would never hear the end of it from Douwe Bergsma, their Chief Marketing Officer. (Through the pandemic he has become a trusted colleague, albeit a fierce competitor too.)

I'm also enormously grateful for all of you. What a time for me to be out! A World Series win (Go Braves!), PR/social media crises, a plane crash, a Magnet conference, and major leadership transitions announced.

You didn't miss a beat. Everything happened smoothly and like clockwork. And, as it should, this is an amazing team!

Thank you for all you did and continue to do,
Amy

⊙ REFLECTION

Inside baseball moment (wink) - we thought about cutting the Maleficent email entry for this book, but as oddball as it is, I insisted on keeping it. Because otherwise, my appendicitis story (and some later posts) would not make sense.

So, here's the unabridged story: Friday's Monster Dash was a premature wash-out, typical for weather-adverse Georgia. It ended up clear by race time. Saturday was both an Atlanta United end-of-season game and an Atlanta Braves' playoff game. As season ticket holders, we went to the soccer game, and I distinctively wore my pearls. There were a lot of people wearing pearls at the United game. For those not in the know, Joc Pederson was on the Atlanta Braves and he just matter-of-fact started wearing a strand of pearls when he played. I first remember noticing them when he was at bat - wait, "is he wearing PEARLS?" Yep, he was. Ridiculous. And that's when I loved him. Those who know me well, know I love the ridiculous. Each birthday I look for ridiculous moments, to celebrate and bring a smile to my face.

The day of the United game, the boys were out, perhaps getting haircuts. I remember having a moment of acid reflux (not normal for me), but there was some leftover rice in the fridge so I ate it and it made me feel better.

We went on to the United game—enjoyed our fried chicken sliders, fries, and wine. By the second half I remember sitting there, when I'm normally rapt, feeling really tired and rundown. It was a literal moment. I shrugged it off and yet I still remember it today.

We got home in time to turn on the Braves game. Had some more wine and am sure the boys made frozen pizza or something. By then my indigestion was mounting - to the point where I went to bed early (on a Saturday!) saying "I'm going to bed, I don't feel well."

I slept a couple hours. But then tossed and turned, super uncomfortable, not sure if I had the flu, a stomach bug or what. I could not get comfortable. I could not sleep. Nothing worked. I finally took my pillow to the living room couch and that didn't work. So I moved to the guest room. Tossed and turned more there, followed by more GI issues on both ends that you don't need to know about.

Normally once the GI issues pass, I feel better, especially in normal circumstances. But I still couldn't relax and sleep. The fever-breaking didn't come; the sweaty but welcome dank dark sleep didn't come. My abdomen and intestines felt hot on the inside. Swollen and on fire.

Finally around 11 am I emerged and told my hubs something wasn't right. It was Halloween and I was supposed to leave the next day to speak at a conference in Vegas.

I texted one of my BFFs, who also had appendicitis and is an MD, to see if I should go to the ED or urgent care. She said the ED because they'd have a CT scanner to confirm diagnosis. Then I texted the CEO of the two closest hospitals to me to see where it was best to go. Afterall it was still pandemic times and I wanted the least wait time.

My husband drove me, dropped me off and went back to help the kiddo with Halloween. I took a glorious Zofran and fluid-fueled nap in the ED and lo and behold - I had appendicitis.

The reason I even went to the ED was because I was supposed to leave for Vegas the next day to speak at my first conference since the pandemic started. The ED doc said it was a good thing I came in because my appendix could've burst in flight!

The Braves played that night with a chance to win the World Series. I remember asking the score of the game when I came out of anesthesia and watching them lose in my recovery room. I got to be home with my family and my parents when they won. My parents came to town to watch Josh because Chris was going to go to Vegas with me. They still came and helped around the house while I was recovering. We even got to watch the whole parade on TV together.

I ended up being out for two weeks. While I probably could have pushed it to go back after a week off, I was simply exhausted. I think more than two years of the pandemic caught up with me physically and emotionally. Perhaps my appendix knew I needed a couple weeks to rest and did me a favor.

✉ **Subject: Making Predictions**

Date: Friday, December 3, 2021, 5:08 p.m.

Team,

In my role, I'm fortunate to be part of several Chief Marketing Officer roundtables, which I've mentioned from time to time. Last night I shared the incredible "quick turn" work this team did in activating the World Series at the Health Marketing Leaders meeting, which is a group of 100 CMOs for health systems across the country. This is the weekly "Rhoda" call that I have referenced where I get lots of great feedback from her and my colleagues sharing how impressed they are with the work that **you** do.

This morning I attended (virtually) Georgia State University's CMO Marketing Roundtable. This is a group of 50+ CMOs from major Atlanta employers, including Truist Bank, Coca-Cola, Delta, Honey Baked Ham, Chick-fil-A, Mercedes-Benz, the Hawks, the Braves, Parkmobile and, more.

This morning's meeting featured a discussion on AI in Marketing with Raj Venkatesan, a professor at the University of Virginia's Darden School of Business. The framework for evaluating and adopting AI in Marketing looks like this:

Acquisition ▶ Retention ▶ Advocacy ▶ Growth
Sound familiar? Raj also posed his definition of marketing, which is:

"Marketing is all about making predictions to deliver the right, best personalized experience."

This definition perfectly captures the critical intersection of science and art needed to succeed in marketing. **It reinforces** my vision for our team's transformation to be acutely data driven, analyzing data to evaluate performance and using data to demonstrate marketing's impact on Emory Healthcare's business objectives. For without strong EBIDA, we cannot improve lives and provide hope.

It also speaks to my long-term vision of making predictions. Ultimately, as we gain more experience and expertise in using data, we can predict and prescribe the number of leads needed to achieve those volume goals. When we can do that, we can model our marketing budget and tactics off budgeted volumes, and then strive to capture those leads at the lowest *effective* cost per acquisition.

I'm curious though: What is your definition of marketing and how does it impact your work and our team?

Our team's marketing transformation continues to amaze and delight me. As the vacant positions on our team fill with wonderful new colleagues like Glen, Miranda, Laura, Jenny and Luis (in January), the momentum is palpable. I am so excited for the calendar year ahead and all that we will accomplish together.

As always, thank you for all you do. I *predict* you will have a wonderful weekend!

Thank you,

Amy

 PRO TIP

Most people are familiar with the acronym "EBITDA," meaning "earnings before interest, taxes, depreciation, and amortization." However, since non-profit organizations, like Emory Healthcare, are tax exempt, we use "EBIDA" which removes the T.

2022

✉ Subject: In Like a Lion

Date: Friday, January 7, 2022, 5:32 p.m.

Well, the new year certainly came in roaring like a lion, didn't it?

When memes have aptly pointed out the homonyms "2022," "2020 too," or "2020 II", I shouldn't have expected anything else. Though I'm sure many of us had hoped for a softer landing.

I can't believe it's only January 7. I feel like I've lived a month in a week's time.

Pandemic living and pandemic working are not for the faint of heart. Especially if your profession happens to be health care.

But how fortunate are we to work in health care at this time?

Sure, we can lament the woes and challenges of being at the very epicenter of the pandemic. But honestly, would you want it any other way? Would you want to be sitting on the sidelines? The outside looking in? Having to make heads or tails of the news reports or social media chatter? I count it a blessing to hear the facts straight from our experts. Does the situation constantly change? Absolutely. However, I know I can count on our incredible infectious disease and epidemiology experts to guide us every step of the way.

That doesn't mean it isn't taxing. It sure can be. Pandemic fatigue is real. The omicron surge — deflating. Colleagues, friends, family or yourself dealing with COVID—worrisome. Accepting the possibility that COVID is just a normal part of life—difficult.

How do we stay resilient? May I offer a few ways:

1. **Perspective**. An easy thing to say, but harder to put into practice. Consider this quote from L. Thomas Holdcroft, *"Life is a grindstone. Whether it grinds us down or polishes us up, depends on us."* Same description, but different outlooks.

2. **Teamwork**. This is an amazing team that accomplishes amazing things. The collaboration is palpable and transformative. I hope you see how far we've come and the results tangible. In Dr. Lewin's own words, *"Marketing has had another exceptional year, and we greatly appreciate the talent and impact that you and your team have demonstrated so conclusively."*

3. **Laughter.** Keep laughing my friends. I love the sense of humor on this team. Laughter truly is the best medicine.

Take some time this weekend to unplug and relax, heal if you are unwell, and laugh a lot.

Thank you for all you do,
Amy

◯ REFLECTION

We rang in the second New Year of pandemic times to the Omicron variant—with the largest amount of recorded cases in U.S. history. Although less deadly, Omicron was highly infectious. In health care we were hit by a double (near triple) pandemic—yet another surge of C+ patients, compounded with many call-outs by health care employees as they fell down with the virus.

In fact, it was this time of year when COVID really hit my team. While one or two had it in the early days of the pandemic, the 2021-2022 holidays hit my team (or their families) especially hard with the virus. We had it at our home too—our son down for the count after going out rollerskating with friends. It was scary. This variant still had the terrible chest congestion and breathing problems. I bought a pulse oximeter to make sure he stayed in range. After a few tenuous days, Josh recovered fairly quickly—the benefit of the fountain of youth.

All of that plus the continued effects of The Great Resignation, made us tired. We didn't enter the new year with a renewed sense of hope and energy, rather a feeling of being on a dreaded hamster wheel of pandemic surges. While around us the world was literally on fire. Wildfires ran rampant throughout Colorado, airlines canceled thousands of flights stranding travelers and rumbles of Russia invading Ukraine. There was no rest for the weary after nearly 20 months of pandemic living.

✉@ **Subject: Clubhouse Rules**

Date: Friday, January 21, 2022, 6:03 p.m.

Hello from Northlake!

The space is shaping up quite nicely. As I told the gang here today, I want to make this space as "Google-esque" as possible. I want Northlake to reflect our team's spirit and be a place we are eager to come to congregate and collaborate.

Apparently, we're already on our way! Patrick's daughter, when she saw our collaboration space a couple weeks ago, said "Oh, this looks like Google! This team must be fun. I want to hang out here." (Patrick is the CEO of our Emory Healthcare Network for those of you who don't know him.)

When I read up on different models for post-pandemic "Return to Office" plans, I immediately gravitated to the **Clubhouse** format. The *HBR*[19] article describes the Clubhouse format as a place for purposeful collaborative work with folks returning to their home offices for focused work.

As humans, we all crave human interaction. As marketers, we need spontaneity. Zoom and Teams do not foster spontaneity. Northlake does.

Today we had a relatively unstructured day that allowed us to connect as individuals, chat and catch up personally, brainstorm ideas for the space, help each other out with small tactical things or work through big ideas.

Like Chuck helping me set up OneDrive and SharePoint on my computer. Or Nikki and I discussing big picture marketing and communication collaboration. Or Cheryl and Glen having lunch at the high-top tables in our break area. Miranda and Glen carefully organizing our supply stations. Denise, Jenny, Miranda, Cheryl and I dreaming ways to set up the collaboration and conference areas to foster connection to our goals, creative and personas.

I cannot wait for Omicron to subside, so we can start collaborating and socializing in our EHC Marketing Clubhouse.

And to all of you, have a wonderful and safe weekend. Hope to see you at Northlake soon.

Thank you,
Amy

 REFLECTION

Our home at Northlake has had so many homecomings. Cheryl had her first job at Northlake. Another colleague who celebrated 32 years with Emory and retired in 2024, talked about how her mom came out of retirement for a customer service role at this mall and was featured in our local papers for her exemplary customer service.

As a Gen Xer, wandering malls and going in and out of stores was our pastime. I remember my mom dropping me off at Boulevard Mall in Buffalo to meet up with a fifth grade friend, where we walked freely around the mall for about an hour. Checking out Claire's, Spencer Gifts and slurping Orange

Julius. It's a weird kind of homecoming for us Gen Xers and Boomers to find ourselves working in an old dilapidated mall—once a place of employment, pastime and joy for us. I'm thankful for Emory, Vanderbilt and other health systems for re-energizing these spaces, and making them vibrant and viable again.

To this day, we love our space at Northlake Mall. Located in a vacated Sears anchor shop. We designed our space to be as collaborative as possible. Every time anyone comes into our marketing space, whether internal Emory or external partners, they love it.

As you now know, Sears and the adjacent vacant Kohl's space were our incredible vaccination site. Nothing in my career will ever compare to that experience. The extreme challenge. The fear. The teamwork. The uncertainty. The exhilaration and the joy of delivering lifesaving vaccines.

Simply the most remarkable time of my career.

✉ **Subject: Yard Sale Lessons**

Date: Friday, January 28, 2022, 6:34 p.m.

Team,

As we reach the end of January (how is this month over already??), I want to share the January 1st reflection from my desk calendar.

Zig Ziglar, author-salesman-marketer-motivational speaker, said **"You don't have to be great at something to start, but you have to start to be great at something."**

Simple, but profound words.

My first start in marketing dates as far back to doing yard sales as a kid to make money for ice cream and skating.

We lived at the corner of Hyledge and High Park Boulevard in Amherst, NY. The two streets met in a perfect T with a dead-end to the left of our house. Hyledge, the top of the T, emptied out onto Eggert Road with High Park leading to Main Street. Both major thoroughfares where I grew up.

The first time I did a yard sale (more like a card table sale in a yard), I put poster board signs at the ends of both streets. I scribbled in crayon something to the effect of **"Yard Sale: Doll Furniture, Doll Clothes, Toys"**. I had little-to-no shoppers.

The next time I changed the sign to: **"Yard Sale: Furniture, Clothes, Toys"** and made the letters as large and readable as possible. Cars and shoppers came streaming by. Some certainly disappointed to see the furniture and clothes were for dolls. But others, impressed by the effort of a 12-year-old girl, bought stuff. I nearly sold out my inventory.

I never became great at yard sales. But I learned my first lesson in marketing that day.

Intrigued by what influences a person to take action, I kept learning and trying new things. In college, I did internships every summer, doing any task asked, soaking up as much as I could. I put that learning to work and continued to hone my craft, working in small non-profits for 10 years. Little by little I got better. Did I have setbacks? Absolutely. But I didn't stop trying or learning. Neither should you.

Fast forward to 2022 and looking back to the 1980s, it's hard to imagine that little girl selling doll furniture is now honored to lead an amazing team of marketers for a nationally recognized health care brand.

I don't profess to be great at marketing; I still have so much to learn and try. In fact, as marketers we can never stop testing and learning. But I did start at something. It lead me to Emory and to all of you: a great team. For that, I'm eternally grateful.

So, with one month of 2022 nearly under our belts, **what do you aspire to be great at and how will you start this year?**

Thank you for all you do,
Amy

✉@ **Subject: Productive or Busy? There's a Difference.**

Date: Friday, February 4, 2022, 4:55 p.m.

Team,

As we close in on the second anniversary of the global pandemic, there's much talk about burnout. We all are feeling it. Yes, me too.

Burnout and overload are not new because of the pandemic. Nor are they unique to health care. Both certainly existed far before, though COVID-19 became an accelerant.

As a team, we have evolved our work and processes to continually address the concern and find better ways to manage our work. That, however, is an imperfect art. Some changes work and some do not. And just when we think we have things under control, another curveball is thrown our way. Such is the nature of health care and marketing.

But... We don't need to let it control us. Rather, we hold the power to control it.

I love analogies and am a sucker for a good inspirational quote. I have been all my life. Next time you are at Northlake ask me to show you the decoupage paper stand that has adorned my work desk since 1994.

Here are a few that remind me, we have the power to change:

First, **"The definition of insanity is doing the same things over and over but expecting a different result."**

- We know this is true. Yet change is hard. And change doesn't always work for the better. However, if we don't try to change, we'll never see different results.

- This year we took a different approach to our planning and budgeting. Portions of it are an incredible success, like the collaboration and an Excel tracker that is a beautiful work of art. Portions, like developing detailed tactical plans and committing budget dollars, not so much. Do I regret the change? Not one minute. We've made improvements and tried something new. We're learning and growing from the successes and the "unsuccesses." FY23 planning will be even better for it.

Second, one of my favorite Walt Disney quotes: **"The way to get started is to quit talking and begin doing."**

- In America, complaining is a competitive sport. While it feels good to vent and get something off our chest, complaining changes absolutely nothing. In fact, it can have a caustic effect, where it makes things worse, instead of better.

- Things only change when we do something different. We do something different, well, by doing something different. This is why you may hear frustration in my voice when we get stuck talking about why or why not, instead of developing a path forward. Change happens when we are deliberate about it. Stop talking, start doing.

Which brings me to my last of the day: **Be Productive, Not Busy.**

- Being busy is a false idol. It makes you feel important. But being busy robs you of Father Time, becoming an excuse or crutch for not taking needed action. Busyness saps our energy, prevents us from focusing on the important stuff, and leaves us feeling empty of accomplishment.

- Being productive, however, is both rewarding and energizing. How satisfied do you feel when you complete a complex and/or important project? When your work has really impacted our business, our team, and better yet, improved lives and provided hope? Being productive produces gratifying results and real change.

So, while there is much for me, our leaders and the organization to address when it comes to burnout, the onus is not on us alone. This is a team sport, and we equally need your commitment and engagement.

When you are feeling burnt out or overloaded, take personal inventory on how you work. Are you being productive or are you being busy? Are you focusing on smaller, easier or less important tasks in the guise of staying "busy"? Or are you focusing on productive work to affect forward progress and real change? When you encounter barriers, raise them on the Huddle board or to your leader. We'll work together to find ways to remove or work around them.

I'm guilty of the Busyness Trap myself. It's easy to take a precious free hour and fill it cleaning up my email, but often that's to the detriment of focused time to analyze campaign and financial performance or do purposeful work on long-term marketing planning. I frequently have to check myself on the Busy-Productive spectrum.

This feels an appropriate moment to dust off our dormant Emory Healthcare tag line: **"We're all in this together."** Overused in the pandemic (we were ahead of our time when we unveiled it in 2013!), it still has meaning. We truly are all in this together.

Only together will we conquer burnout. Only together will we grow. **Only together are we a team.**

As always, thank you for all you do,
Amy

✉ Subject: Curveball

Date: Friday, February 18, 2022, 5:59 p.m.

Team,

Two weeks ago, I wrote: *"And just when we think we have things under control, another curveball is thrown our way."*

I didn't expect we'd be pitched one so soon.

This curveball comes in the form of our own staffing challenges.

The departures of three marketing colleagues, two teammates on FMLA, and another's promotion to another team have dropped our capacity by nearly 25%.

How quickly things can change, as just last month, we celebrated being nearly fully staffed, enjoying the energy and excitement our new teammates Jenny, Miranda, Luis and Laura bring.

No doubt this curveball sucked some of the wind from our sails.

While we are excited for our colleagues as they grow their careers, and wish our other colleagues good health and speedy recovery, it no doubt presents yet another hurdle to leap.

But where do we find the energy? With each new hurdle, we have to reach deeper into our reserves, hoping there is some energy left. Sometimes there isn't.

It's okay to feel frustrated and exhausted. But we cannot wallow.

Continuing the baseball analogy, we have to step back up to the plate. Yet instead of standing there, letting curveballs whiz by and striking out, we need to hit that curveball. It doesn't need to be a home run. Simply hitting a single off that curve is forward progress. As we saw with our championship-winning Braves, sometimes it's small ball that wins the game.

A poignant article from *Harvard Business Review*[20] discusses our current psychological phase of the pandemic. Please take the time to read it. I hope you find it resonates.

As the author notes, ***"we're all walking wounded,"*** and as the title states we *"need time to rehabilitate"* from the pandemic. It is important to acknowledge this. Admit it to ourselves. Say it out loud. For once we name it, we can face it.

I like the prescription the author gives for managing through this phase:

1. **Don't move too fast.** (We cannot solve for everything at once)
2. **Value progress.** (Huddle kudos, EHC Recognize and celebrating the Greens in Traffic are important)
3. **Have compassion.** (Akin to Dane's pandemic mantra of having Grace and Patience for ourselves and each other)

We will get through this. One step at a time, little by little, soon we'll find our tanks full again. And we'll be hitting those curveballs out of the park.

Thank you for all you do,
Amy

⊙ REFLECTION

Today is January 29, 2024, and this was my last reflection to write. Truthfully, I've been avoiding it. Not because it is the last one I needed to write, but because it's the hardest. Author David Rock said, "We're all walking wounded." This is especially true for those of us in health care who acutely and viscerally experienced the pandemic. We *never* had time to rehabilitate—still haven't in my humble opinion.

First the adrenaline and odd excitement of a new foe and sheltering in place for eight weeks. Then eight months until the hope of a vaccine emerged. Then eight more weeks of vaccine distribution and shortage insanity. Followed by a brief eight-week relief—the summer of 2021 was glorious— we all thought the pandemic was *over*! Only to come back to another freaking surge. More ups and downs and hello Omicron in 2022. And the Great Resignation, which *Wikipedia* says started March 2021 and ended June 2023.

How on Earth does one, in health care, find the resilience to keep bouncing back from all of this? Seriously. We all need a sabbatical. But even with each vacation and dutiful PTO, we come back to more of the same. It's nearly impossible to get ahead of it. To dig deep and find a new way out.

I've likened this whole experience to what I call health care's "Blockbuster Moment."[21] We are experiencing incredible and traumatic industry disruption. But we cannot fail. If we fail, it means failing society. Failing our loved ones, the health of our communities, ourselves.

We are not Blockbuster. We cannot shutter our doors and leave one remaining artifact in an obscure part of the country. We treat people's lives. Yet, in Blockbuster's case, where Netflix became the new way to consume content without leaving your house, health care doesn't work the same way.

The drop in telehealth visits as the pandemic waned is proof positive. People need people. Sick people need doctors and nurses. IRL. While telehealth and virtual care are amazing things that help to increase access, at the end of the day they do not replace in-person care. Telehealth cannot do cancer infusions. It cannot perform microvascular decompression brain surgery. It cannot place a stent, deliver a baby, place an IUD, or treat an ear fungus.

No, we can't quit, but we're up against all odds. The financial model, the reimbursement model, the layers of bureaucracy and regulation and all the things I know are meant to keep us safe, keep adding more cost and burnout to the health care industry in America. All of this while fewer Americans are choosing health care as a career. Can I blame them? No. But what will come of us all when the entire system breaks?

And so, four years later. I'm exhausted. I'm spent. Doing yoga to find inner calm to make my way through each new challenge.

But no one wants to listen. No one wants to hear about our struggles. Everyone has moved on, but us. But we cannot. Heart attacks, strokes, births, cancers, menopause, aging—they don't quit.

Four long years later, the road is long and tough.

I've had team members go out on FMLA for burnout. I know I've lost others to burnout who resigned. While I appreciate the need to rebound, I feel like the rubber band you find in the way back of your junk drawer. Once resilient, but now hard, dried up and brittle. How did this happen? Slowly over time. Just as the Grand Canyon was carved artfully over years and years of abrasion.

And if I'm this exhausted as a health care marketer, what about the rest of the health care workforce?

Subject: Agape Love

Date: Friday, March 4, 2022, 5:17 p.m.

Team,

Clearly I was "in my feelings" about the war on Ukraine during staff meeting Monday. Thank you for allowing me the space to express myself. I appreciate your sharing your own personal connections, observations and concerns as well.

In the days since, in addition to becoming more distraught (i.e. nuclear power plant, Africans and Asians facing challenges in evacuating), I've read a good bit about how this war is getting more attention than other equally as disturbing conflicts: Afghanistan, Syria, Rwanda, South Sudan, and countless others. Even the less traditional, but no less devastating, wars on drugs, guns, domestic terrorism and racial inequity here in our own country.

When I step back, I see they emanate from the same place. Someone thinking they are better than someone else. Their avarice, ego and hunger for power taking such precedence, they are willing to commit violent and dangerous acts to prove their point.

A student of Dr. King and Gandhi, I believe there is no place for violence. Violence only begets more violence. Agape love however allows for kindness and discord to co-exist. It channels our energy in the right direction and frees us from the burden of hatred.

But agape love is not always easy. We cannot eliminate conflict. We can, however, choose how we respond to it. I have spent my life as a consensus-builder. No doubt I get frustrated with conflict, but instead of bulldozing my way across, I do my best to seek to understand.

Processing conflict this way takes more time. Some may say it is not taking a hard enough stand on issues. But the reality is, if we don't seek to understand others, we'll never find common ground. We won't progress.

As Ginni Rometty, former CEO of IBM, said: "Growth and comfort do not co-exist." To this I agree, and further offer that agape love gives us the foundation to grow through our discomfort.

Take a moment to hear Dr. King[22] himself explain agape love. I hope you find it resonates. Wishing peace for Ukraine, and peace for us all,
Amy

✉@ **Subject: The fabric of our lives**

Date: Friday, March 11, 2022, 5:31 p.m.

Team,

Can you believe it? Today marks the two year anniversary of the coronavirus global pandemic. COVID-19 still here among us.

Out of curiosity I looked up the traditional second anniversary gift: Cotton.

How very fitting, isn't it?

As the pandemic moves into endemic phase, we now know the virus is unlikely to disappear completely. So we learn to live with it. The fabric of our lives. We persevere and evolve as humans do. But the thread of COVID is always there. Woven into our minds, our lives, our way of life.

But just like the threat of terrorism in the wake of September 11 didn't stop us from living and thriving, neither should the threat of COVID-19. It gets less and less deadly with each variant. And thanks to discoveries by scientists at academic medical centers across the world, including Emory, we know how to treat it. To snuff it out—whether preventatively through vaccines and Evusheld[23], curatively through molnupiravir[24], remdesivir[25], or monoclonal antibodies, or attentively through careful and compassionate expert care at the bedside.

To this day, 20,758 people are living thanks to the attentive care they received in our hospitals—a global best 93% survival rate. Countless more who received curative care in our outpatient settings. And never forget the nearly 200,000 Georgians we helped vaccinate. If this isn't improving lives and providing hope, I don't know what is.

So while coronavirus is not a comfy white cotton T-shirt I ever want to wear, I suppose it can be part of the fabric of our lives. We've proven we can live, move, and, dare I say, thrive among it.

Thank you for all you do,
Amy

Subject: Happy Holi

Date: March 18, 2022, 4:45 p.m.

Team,

Yesterday was St. Patrick's Day, but did you know today is Holi[26]?

This morning while checking my calendar to start my day, I noticed my holiday notification said Holi. It came up again in conversation with Cheryl and Laura over lunch at Northlake. I didn't know much about it, so did a little online research to learn more.

Known as the festival of colors, Holi welcomes spring and celebrates the triumph of good over evil. Holifestival.org[27] further explains the legends "associated with Holi reassure the people the power of the truth . . . is the ultimate victory of good over evil."

As we've passed the two-year mark of the pandemic, I cannot help but make the connection to science. Science—especially truth in science—has been our beacon, our guiding light giving us hope and leading us through the pandemic. We did not always have the answers, but we always knew we could trust in science.

Looking back, science helped us battle the evil of an invisible virus that swept the globe, infecting millions and taking far too many lives. Yet science prevailed: treatments, discoveries and vaccines bringing us victory over that evil.

Take a moment to read about Holi[28] and spend some time celebrating the arrival of spring, the weakening of the coronavirus and the eternal hope that good will always prevail over evil.

Happy Holi,
Amy

✉ **Subject: Plunging into the swirl**

Date: Friday, March 25, 2022, 4:31 p.m.

Team,

Today I heard a Taoist fable that really resonated. It goes like this:

"An old man was walking along a river. He lost his balance and accidentally fell into the river rapids. Those rapids led to a very high and dangerous waterfall. Onlookers feared for his life. Yet, miraculously, he emerged alive and unharmed, albeit soaking wet, at the end of the falls. When asked how he managed to survive. He said **'I accommodated myself to the water, not the water to me. Without thinking, I allowed myself to be shaped by it. Plunging into the swirl, I came out with the swirl. This is how I survived.'"**

Those who know me well, know that I believe the key to success, in your career, in life, in marketing, and especially at Emory, is adaptability.

We work in an ecosystem. An ecosystem that has a constant current. Emory's current may change as our environment changes, but it is always constant and fast flowing. If we are not careful, we can get caught up in the rapids and find ourselves plunging over the dangerous waterfall.

Just as you cannot change the force of rapids in a river, nor can you change Emory's current. It may ebb and flow, but it never goes away. So how do we find success like the old man in the fable and accommodate ourselves to our waters? Further, how do we allow ourselves to be shaped by it to not only survive it, but master it?

I have been whitewater rafting twice in my life—down the Hudson River in the Adirondack mountains. The first time was the most exhilarating. Our guide took us down the river swiftly and expertly.

Amazingly we were among the first back, though we were not among the first to go. We thought we were just really good rafters, speedily beating everyone else. Instead, we learned that our boat had a slow leak!

And that leak was on my side of the boat. Sitting front left in the raft, I didn't notice anything. But my husband noticed it. By the end of the two-and-a-half hour journey, I was visibly lower than the rest of my family. Fortunately I never fell out, though I did get a wicked sunburn.

Clearly, our guide saw this happening. He didn't say a word, but calmly and expertly navigated our complete journey down the river, through the rapids and over waterfalls. He ensured we had an amazing experience, but also made sure to deliver us safely back to land.

Neither Hudson River nor our leaky raft accommodated us, but our guide accommodated the situation.

After nearly 18 years of living in and studying the Emory ecosystem, I consider myself a pretty good guide.

It hasn't always come easy. I've had my fair share of capsizing, falling overboard, dodging boulders and ungracefully tumbling down waterfalls. But I always got back into the boat. Learned from those experiences, how to recognize turbulent water, navigate around the bends, plunge into the swirl and emerge alive—often stronger for it.

Each of you too is learning Emory. Some days you may capsize, but that's okay, it's all part of the experience. When that happens, hold on to the float and let your teammates lift you back up to safety.

Back in the boat, you start again, another journey, another trek down the exhilarating river. Rinse and repeat, as Denise would say. Until suddenly you'll find you too are an expert guide—with your own stories to tell. Your own successes. Your own pitfalls. Growing your own Emory wisdom.

Together, we are stronger for our collective wisdom. It gives us the power to survive the swirl—and perhaps find exhilaration in it too.

Thank you for all you do,
Amy

✉ Subject: Holy Celebration Coincidence

Date: Friday, April 15, 2022, 5:42 p.m.

Team,

While Easter and Passover often overlap in the spring, this year is unique. Again, very on brand for 2022!

Today Good Friday falls on the first night of Passover. And both fall in the middle of Ramadan, which is a rare occurrence.[29]

I enjoyed reading Dr. Khan's message[30] about Ramadan, and read a little more, just now, about the similarities between Easter and Passover[31].

Growing up in a community with many Catholic and Jewish families, I'm reminded again of the similarities (as well as differences) between our religions. And it's no surprise to see the overlap of the Old Testament, New Testament and Torah in these celebrations.

There were not many Muslims in my suburb of Buffalo, N.Y., so I didn't know much about Ramadan. I loved learning about the daily fasting and the daily break-fast celebrations. Further fascinated to read Dr. Khan's insight that many professional athletes find Ramadan a time of peak performance. Perhaps the intermittent fasting fad might possibly emulate Ramadan or even emanate from it?

I'm also struck by the levels of fasting, abstention and intentional deprivation common among all three rituals. And, most of all, the celebrations of freedom, life, and love they all represent. Whether you are Christian, Jewish, Muslim, another faith, or don't follow a religion, I know we can all agree that celebrating life and love is a good thing.

To those that celebrate, I wish you:

Happy Easter
Joyous and Kosher Passover
Ramadan Mubarak

And to all—enjoy your weekend,
Amy

📧 Subject: Earth Day Gratitude

Date: Friday, April 22, 2022, 5:04 p.m.

Team,

Today is Earth Day. But rather than share some insights and research on the meaning of the day, I'd like to share my gratitude for a special person in my life still being on Earth—my husband, Chris.

Twelve years ago today we were still in the Neuro ICU at Emory University Hospital, the fourth day after his brain surgery.

On April 19, 2010 Dr. Boulis performed microvascular decompression (MVD) to relieve Chris' trigeminal neuralgia (TN). TN is a compression of the trigeminal nerve that creates electric like shocks through your head and face at random.

TN came out of the blue. He was perfectly fine and then one day in 2009 started having symptoms. We spent months with many different specialists at Emory figuring out what was going on— PCP, ENT, Neuro. Eventually confirming our worst fear that Dr. Google's diagnosis of TN was correct.

After rounds of other treatments and various medications that didn't work or caused other unbearable symptoms, we made the decision to have brain surgery. I was in business school and Josh was not even in kindergarten yet. It was a scary and hectic time for us. The biggest decision we ever had to make.

I'll never forget sitting in the surgery waiting room calmly on the outside, but a nervous wreck on the inside. Family and friends helped me through. And my Emory colleagues in marketing, radiology, and former university colleagues served as a tremendous support.

A few hours later Dr. Boulis called me to say the surgery was a success and that Chris had a lot of stuff wound around his trigeminal nerve causing the issue. Boulis padded it all up, put a plate in my husband's head, and moved him to post-op.

Chris stayed in post-op, and I was in the waiting room, for a long time. The Neuro ICU was full with other patients and there was no room for him to move to. Eventually they moved him to a room on the Cardiac ICU, where I joined him. A long night, but so relieved to see him emerge successfully from the surgery. We moved to the Neuro ICU the next day and remained there until discharge on April 23.

Recovery was not without its challenges, and we had no idea what the road ahead would bring.

It's remarkable to be at year 12, far past the five-year success rate of the surgery. And life is **normal**.

We survived brain surgery, a global pandemic and are surviving raising a teenager.

Each year we celebrate Chris' "Brainniversary" in a dull and normal fashion: with wine and takeout food. This year it was Thai and Malbec.

I don't need to tell you that I'm a firm believer in science. We all are, or else, we wouldn't be working in health care.

But every day, and especially this Earth Day, I am thankful for science, medicine, discovery, innovation and the incredible team at Emory Healthcare that gave us normal back. For that I'm forever grateful.

We work for an amazing organization that does truly life-saving work, including my own (thank you appendix) and my husband's. Thanks for allowing me to share my testimony with you.

Happy Earth Day and celebrate being "above the grass, instead of below it" as my Dad always says.

Thank you,
Amy

✉️ **Subject: Potential**

Date: Friday, April 29, 2022, 5:40 p.m.

Team,

"Our potential is one thing. What we do with it is quite another," said author Angela Duckworth. It is so apropos that my daily inspirational quote calendar featured her words yesterday.

She perfectly captures how far we've transformed Emory Healthcare's marketing strategy, as evidenced in last night's Marketing Executive Advisory Committee meeting.

Those of you in attendance heard our leaders laud our efforts. We've clearly demonstrated there is a science to marketing, as much as there is an art to it.

I always knew we had this potential and to see it come to fruition brings me great joy.

Little known fact: my parents arrived yesterday at 3:45 p.m. for an overnight stay on their Snow Bird migration back to Buffalo.

When I finally closed my computer at 6:10 p.m., and joined my family, my mom asked me what the meeting was and how it went. As I started describing the meeting, who attends and what we've accomplished, I had to pause. As I sat there, thought about it and tried to describe it to someone who really doesn't get what I do, I simply said: "It's really a big deal. Really big." Going on to say it is the culmination of years of hard work and rewarding to see my vision and lifelong career goal come into full view.

Although it made for a hectic day, I'm glad my parents were here. I'm glad my mom asked me that question, because otherwise I might not have taken that pause to reflect on all we've accomplished.

We have done something quite special and our future is bright. I cannot wait to see where our collective potential takes us next.

Thank you for all you do,
Amy

REFLECTION

This MEAC (Marketing Executive Advisory Committee) meeting was all about *data*. We shared insights from our first two years of CRM data: 186 campaigns and micro-campaigns led to over 28,000 leads, $12 million in direct marketing-influenced contribution margin and $70 million of indirect marketing-influenced contribution margin. Direct means the revenue is directly attributable to the campaign, while indirect means the full amount of that leads to impact on the system post capture.

Direct means the reveenue is directly attributable to the campaign, while indirect means the patient came to us through a direct marketing tactic, but then went on to utilize different services. And then we showed how we'd use this data to inform our FY23 marketing strategy—doubling down on low cost, high-value work like location listings, paid search, and experimenting more with email and marketing automation.

✉ Subject: Micro-tears

Date: Friday, May 20, 2022, 6:43 p.m.

Team,

When I turned 49 last year, I embarked on a journey to become "Fit by 50".

I was making pretty good progress hitting my lowest weight since my carefree twenties in October and beginning to build lean muscle mass. Alas, my surprise Halloween appendectomy waylaid those plans and I found myself losing all that progress when I got on the scale last month.

So, I re-committed to my "Fit by 50" plan and got back on my fitness routine: brisk walks for mental and physical health, and weight training through an online program. After a month of diligent work, I wasn't seeing the scale nor my measurements move much.

I started Dr. Googling and learned about micro-tears[32].

These are small tears in the muscle from working out, especially weight training, that are completely normal and needed to build lean muscle mass. Inflammation and fluid retention[33] are also a normal part of the muscle's healing process. As a result, people who start new exercise programs, tend to retain more water while the muscles adjust to their new environment and skill set. This means the scale doesn't move as fast as one would like at first, but eventually it does. (Well, let's hope so at least!)

Why am I telling you this?

It's not to encourage you to start your own fitness routine—although self-care is very important! Rather, as I continue to read about micro-tears, it makes me think a lot about the transition our team is going through.

In addition to bandwidth challenges from our vacancies, we are in the midst of our own new workout routine. One that has us learning and building new marketing muscle mass and muscle memory.

From our exciting Gap Fill drip campaign, including today's "go/ no go" session, to building and using new analytics capabilities, to customized "Emory Near You" emails, to our monthly editorial meetings and developing new ways to collaborate on content, to this year's all-digital Community Health Needs Assessment process and even continuing to hone our project management and budget chops—we've got a lot of Marketing "weight training" going on!

Form is equally important. Make sure you are mastering your form before you add more weight to your routine, otherwise you risk injury. In the case of marketing muscle, that could take many forms. Start with a pilot or hypothesis to test. Build one campaign flowchart or one lead nurturing campaign to start. Otherwise, you may risk your own "marketing injury," like skipping a step in the process and finding a tactic deploys with a typo, broken link or incorrect CTA.

We are no doubt each experiencing our own "micro-tears" in our continued marketing evolution. When you're feeling the effects of a "marketing micro-tear," don't give up.

Understand where you are feeling it and why. Allow your body and mind to process the change, but don't stop your new exercise routine. Keep at it—those micro-tears are making us stronger. And as a result, making our patients and community healthier.

The opportunity to transform Emory Healthcare's marketing and patient engagement to the next level is palpable and thrilling. May we continue with our new routine, continuing to learn, grow and experiment. Soon we'll look in the mirror to admire our new buff marketing muscles and find we're the fittest marketing team of all.

Thank you for all you do,
Amy

Subject:On COVID & Juneteenth

Date: Friday, June 17, 2022, 5:26 p.m.

Team,

This week has given me a lot to reflect on—COVID and Juneteenth.

On COVID

Recovering from COVID has given me a new appreciation for science, discovery and innovation. I am awed by the power of a virus to evolve and create new variants. I am ever thankful for vaccines and having access to them. And I recognize the privilege I have in the ability to work from home though this recovery, whereas our clinical colleagues, teachers and other professions cannot.

While my case is mild, it definitely packs a punch. The fatigue is real. I share great empathy to those of you who survived COVID ahead of me—please accept my apology for not fully understanding what you experienced at the time. And for those of you who lost loved ones to COVID, like my husband's uncle, please accept my deepest sympathy.

On Juneteenth

As I shared last year, I had only recently learned about Juneteenth and committed to continuing to learn more and to being part of the solution. This week, toward that end, I watched Power to Heal[34]. In short, it has changed my life.

I had no idea that Medicare[35] was created with intent to provide equity in health care. Medicare is directly related to the desegregation of hospitals, not only in the South, but across the entire country.

On yesterday's panel, Emory's own Dr. Nanette Wenger[36], the Godmother of cardiology, spoke about what it was like when she arrived in Atlanta in the 1950s, saying "Racism was the law of the land."

She went on to talk about how much progress had been made in the years since—Atlanta and her patient base are incredibly diverse. Illustrating the point by sharing she uses the "language line five to six times" a day to speak with her patients in their native languages.

Yet, as we all know, we have so far still to go. She spoke passionately about social determinants of health and the urgent need to address issues of access, quality care, safety, fresh food and integrating health into our education system. At age 91, she is a dynamo! A true living legend—who still speaks, advocates and sees patients.

Thank you for all you do,
Amy

📩 **Subject: Dreambuilders**

Date: Friday, July 22, 2022, 5:44 p.m.

Team,

As I've mentioned in talking with many of you this week, my mantra for FY23 is "Stop Talking, Start Doing." And, we're doing just that.

While Meeting-Free July probably hasn't felt very meeting-free to you, what it has done is free up the time and space to focus on FY23 planning. That is one of the primary reasons EHC implemented Meeting-Free July.

Together we have embraced the spirit of continuous improvement, keeping the good from last year's planning process, identifying the gaps, and closing them. I hope you are seeing how a construct like Lean and EmPower can help us assess, plan and move things forward in a methodical, logical and (mostly) objective way.

Lee Iacocca[37], well-known Chrysler CEO, said: "The discipline of writing something down is the first step toward making it happen."

When we write down our ideas, wishes, gaps, challenges, hopes and dreams, we give them credence. We give ourselves a way to process, sort and prioritize them. And in some cases, dismiss or defer them, so they no longer take up space or hold us back from progress on the others.

In the System ADD workgroup that Chuck and I co-chair, we are finally writing down the things we have talked about for years.

We're analyzing them, sorting them and proposing solutions. The "writing down" is the first step of our "Stop Talking" and the beginning of our "Start Doing." While it takes time and effort, the work is energizing. We are seeing ways to solve and visualize issues that have plagued our department for years.

I hope your planning efforts are bearing the same fruit and energizing you in similar ways. I'm looking forward to bringing it all together on Tuesday.

Four years ago, at exactly 3:23 p.m. on September 30, 2018 (thank you iPhotos for the time stamp), I saw a sign walking through EPCOT. It drives me daily—providing inspiration or a nudge to move things forward. It is the source of my mantra.

"Stop Talking, Start Doing."

I look forward to continuing to build our dreams with this amazing team.

Thank you for all you do,
Amy

✉@ **Subject: Control what you can control**

Date: Friday, July 29, 2022, 5:25 p.m.

Team,

I've been reflecting on our discussion on Tuesday. With so much disruption in our industry and real challenges within our own organization, it's hard not to fall into the "swirl." In the midst of all of this, how do we truly *stop talking and start doing*?

I love dealing with and trying to solve complex problems.

As a kid, I looked forward to the arrival of *GAMES* magazine[38] in the mail, eager to complete every page. Logic problems and eyeball benders my favorites. Pretty sure I was the only one in my tenth grade geometry class that loved solving tautologies[39]. Fast forward to grad school in 2009, I found odd joy in Jeff Rummel's[40] Data and Decision Analysis class.

Given all this, solving for FY23 should be right up my alley. So why is it so difficult?

Then it dawned on me, I thrive on logic. Logic, and a process for working through it, helps me find my way. Yet the problem our industry is facing is so vastly complex, I'm not sure there is a logical way to process ourselves out of it. But sitting in the swirl doesn't help us either.

This has left me doing a lot of thinking, and I think best while walking. So, Wednesday I went for a walk in the neighborhood, popping in my earbuds, and turning to some podcasts. After listening to Denise's fabulous interview on Formstack's podcast, I selected an option from HBR's Coaching Real Leaders podcast. [41]

The episode featured executive coach Muriel Wilkins[42] working with a leader trying to get his confidence back. The crux of the matter is the difference between *focusing on the outcome vs. focusing on the process*. When we focus on the outcome, we're focusing on something in the future, something we cannot control.

She gave this very astute example relating this to sports (and you all know I love a good sports analogy!):

"MURIEL WILKINS: Okay. Let me use an example for you. I have a kid who plays competitive sports and if you've ever played a competitive sport, of course you want to win. But in reality, the only thing you can control is how you play the game, not necessarily the outcome. **We've seen some of the most amazing athletes get on a court, get on a field, wanting to win. That's the desired outcome, but they can't really control the outcome because the outcome is in the future. The only thing they can control is what's happening in the here and now, which is how they play the game.** In your case, how you play the game is this learning and mastering what is necessary to increase the probability of you getting that next role. But it doesn't guarantee that you will get the next role. So why place your confidence on something that's a variable that's not guaranteed, that can be a moving target, that may not even be fully defined yet? Place your confidence, your belief in yourself in the things that you can control. And so what are the things that you can control?"

Sound familiar?

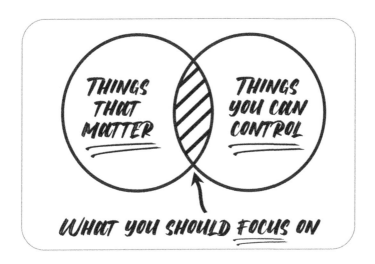

It's the Venn diagram we used in our June planning session to help sort and prioritize our work for the year. One thing is 100% certain: fixing the website is in our control and something that matters. And only Marketing can do it. So that becomes priority #1. Decision made.

Balancing Talent Acquisition and Patient Acquisition, Retention and Loyalty depend on variables that we cannot control. Both are extremely important to the organization, but we have to approach them from the lens of what we can control and what only Marketing can do.

So when we get into the swirl, focus back on what we can control, and we'll find the path ahead clears.

Thank you for all you do,
Amy

✉ Subject: Second Chance

Date: Friday, August 5, 2022, 5:35 p.m.

Team,

Monday marked the start of our 2022-23 Rockdale County school year, and with it resumed my "car rides with Josh," listening to different artists each day from his playlists. Only difference now, he's the one driving so he can rack up the 40 hours he needs to take his driver's test.

Yesterday's feature? T-Pain.

Josh and I are both big T-Pain fans. We have listened to his music a LOT together. Even tried to catch his Road to Wiscansin tour earlier this year. Unfortunately Josh's soccer schedule kept us from the Atlanta show and we couldn't figure out a way to get to any of his out-of-state concerts.

Yesterday, "Second Chance (Don't Back Down)"[43] came on from T-Pain's *Oblivion* album. Though I've heard the song before, it particularly struck me yesterday. So much so that I asked Josh to play it again this morning.

I absolutely LOVE the harmonies. But it's the lyrics that stopped me this time around:

> **"That's no way to live"**
> **"Shut down in my very own backyard"**
> **"I've just played with the hand they deal us"**
> **"Where you couldn't even pay to get away from the pain"**
> **"I've been down for too many days"**

and then into the final chorus and verse:

> **"In this crazy world, we all deserve a second chance**
> **In this crazy world, we all deserve a second chance**
> **Don't back down, don't back down, not now, not never**
> **Who better to fix you other than you? ooh**
> **You know exactly what you want, you know exactly what**
> **you gotta do**
> **You just gotta do it, do it**
> **You just gotta do it, do it"**

Now T-Pain wrote this in 2017, three years before the pandemic, with clear poignancy from his own life experiences.

But I couldn't help draw an emotional parallel to our lives since COVID-19 changed our world in 2020, particularly as health care workers. While the day-to-day toil of fighting the coronavirus pandemic may be over, pandemic fatigue still lingers. That fatigue further burdened by the industry disruption and seemingly insurmountable workforce crisis we find ourselves in.

Say what?? Did she just try to connect T-Pain to health care?? You bet. Think about it:

- **"That's no way to live"**—Shelter-in-place, endless quarantines
- **"Shut down in my very own backyard"**—Shelter-in-place, endless quarantines
- **"I've just played with the hand they deal us"**—Dealing with vaccine shortages and ever changing eligibility rules, COVID surges, making the most of our limited marketing budget dollars and resources, even responding to Monkeypox this week

- **"Where you couldn't even pay to get away from the pain"**—Pandemic fatigue, the Great Resignation, industry disruption
- **"I've been down for too many days"**—All of it gets to the best of us

But. . . **in this crazy world, we all deserve a second chance. Don't back down, not now, not never.**—Yes, we do and it speaks to our resilience and drive as a team.

Who better to fix you other than you?—Sound familiar? Right, focus on what you can control.

You know exactly what you want, you know exactly what you gotta do. You just got do it, do it.—Yes we do. Stop talking, start doing.

If **Stop talking, Start doing** is my FY23 Mantra, **Second Chance (Don't Back Down)** just might be my theme song for FY23.

We know what to do, so let's go do it!

Thank you for all you do,
Amy

P.S. Josh will either be completely mortified or really impressed that T-Pain made it to my Friday email. Hard to tell.

P.P.S. After 30-40 minutes of searching the Google wormhole, I couldn't find T-Pain's story behind the song. If any of you know, please fill me in.

P.P.P.S. Did you know that he collaborated with an Italian composer and pianist on this piece? Check out Roberto Cacciapaglia.

✉ Subject: Patience is a Virtue
Date: Friday, August 19, 2022, 5:07 p.m.

I confess to being impatient this week. Known for my calm demeanor, I don't like being impatient. But it happens to the best of us.

The industry disruption, our workforce challenges, the flip of the fiscal, and the FY23 demand for marketing exceeding our resources (both labor and financial) contributors to that impatience.

Ironically, yesterday I heard a story about patience and it gave me a fresh perspective.

The narrator offered that impatience is a choice.

When we feel ourselves become impatient we can either fill with stress or remain calm. If we choose impatience, there will "always be a correlating body stressor." I'd argue there are times when the body or mind stressor presents itself first which creates a visceral impatient reaction. I imagine both are true.

The key however is to recognize impatience, acknowledge it, and then choose how you wish to deal with it. If you choose stress, you accept the reaction. If you chose calm, you also accept the reaction. It's a matter of which reaction is healthiest for you.

The story ended with this quote: **"Being patient means that rather than stressing out about things we can't rush or change, we use that time to enjoy our life."**

Focusing on "things we can't rush or change," again rings familiar.

We are wasting our breath and energy focusing and stressing on things we cannot control.

We can and should, however, focus on the things we can control, especially those that matter. For me, in this case, that means patience and impatience are acceptable reactions, if it helps get ourselves to our goal. Sometimes impatience is the jolt needed to get something over the finish line.

But if that impatience is directed at something we cannot change or control, it creates unnecessary stress. Nobody needs, and certainly nobody wants, unnecessary stress.

Patience may not be easy, but it is a virtue. And when practiced well, it provides the clarity to focus your energy on things that both matter and that you can control.

As we close out the week, I wish you a weekend free from stress and impatience and one full of enjoying life.

Thank you for all you do,
Amy

Subject: Ruthless Prioritization

Date: Friday, August 26, 2022, 3:16 p.m.

Team,

Prioritize ruthlessly.

In turbulent times, like a global pandemic or industry disruption, setting priorities and maintaining focus on them are critical. Anything else is a distraction that keeps you from your goal.

In yesterday's MEAC meeting, I used the guidance our executive leadership team gave EHC leaders in January to layout our FY23 marketing recommendations.

This guidance specifically outlined five leadership principles from Captain "Sully" Sullenberger[44], the pilot that safely landed his plane in the Hudson River in 2009.

I focused on the first two: **"Prioritize Ruthlessly"** and **"Determine and Decide."**

Our system's marketing demands outstrip the available resources, both labor and dollars. A classic economic principle[45]. Therefore, we must prioritize our work for greatest impact. Focusing on that which only Marketing can control to achieve what is important to Emory Healthcare's success.

In reviewing the FY23 AOP, it is abundantly clear that our number one priority is the website. This is not a job just for our TechOps team, it is a job for every single one of us on the Marketing team. Second is Epic. These two items must rise to the top of our priority list to achieve system objectives.

Web will be a year-long effort. Epic, hopefully, short-lived.

Once we get through Epic, we can move on to the next priorities: Gap Fill and Demand Generation. I will continue to work with leadership to ruthlessly prioritize in order to swiftly determine and decide our priorities for demand generation.

Only with this ruthless prioritization can we achieve our goals. Anything that gets in the way must be put on the Huddle board so it can be escalated.

While the demands can feel burdensome, ruthless prioritization will provide the clarity and space we need to achieve our goals.

If you haven't seen it, take 12 minutes out of your day to watch Captain Sully describe the events of that day[46] and how he put these principles to work.

Thank you for all you do,
Amy

✉ Subject: A little oomph

Date: Friday, September 23, 2022, 5:34 p.m.

Team,

Check out this quote I came across this week:

"The difference between try and triumph is a little 'umph.'"

This is not one I've heard before, but I love it. Growing, improving, tackling projects big and small requires work. Sometimes it's that extra oomph or "umph" that not only gets you over the finish line, but makes a lasting impact.

Can you think of a time when a little oomph made a big difference in your life?

I can think of several on the personal and professional fronts. Professionally, an oomph landed me my first job at Emory University in 2004. Many of you know that music and the performing arts were my first industry. I knew it would take convincing to switch industries, so I did a heck of a lot of research and preparation for my series of interviews leading up to my hire. I even prepared a leave-behind folder with samples of work I would do if I were in the role, including drafting a weekly email of newsworthy tidbits from the school I'd send to the media. I learned months after landing the job that leave-behind is what rose me to their top choice. That extra "umph" lead to triumph.

Personally, I almost didn't accept a role coaching my youngest sister's softball team. The league manager approached me and a friend of mine, since we played on our high school varsity team and had played many years in the Connie Mack league. They'd never had female nor teenager coaches before, but felt we would do a great job given we were active players. Adele and I almost didn't do it because we'd never coached before and were nervous about it. We took a chance and went for it. Putting all the "oomph" into it that we had, especially against skeptical parents who are used to dads as coaches. Long story short, it was a fairy tale ending. We ended up winning the championship against the most winningest, most competitive and most skeptical dad coach of them all. Another series of umphs that literally lead to triumph. My sister said it was her favorite year playing.

And here at Emory Healthcare, our marketing team has too many umphs to count! Just look at all the progress we've made over the years and the incredible impact you have had on improving lives and providing hope.

I'd love to hear your "umph to triumph" story!

Thanks for all you do,
Amy

✉️ **Subject: Fresh Beginning**

Date: Friday, September 30, 2022, 5:56 p.m.

Team,

Two years whizzed by. I can hardly believe we are on the eve of our Epic go-live. From the very start, we knew it was the single biggest and single best thing we could do to improve access for our patients.

We knew it wouldn't be easy, and it wasn't. It has taken a LOT of hard work, systemness and focus to get here. While we play a small part in the technical configuration and implementation, we play the most major part in telling our patients about it.

I am so proud of how this team came together, rolled up your virtual sleeves, and did what needed to be done to let 1.2 million Emory patients know that a fresh beginning is ahead.

Will the near road ahead be rocky? No doubt. But the light at the end of this Epic tunnel shines brightly.

As patients ourselves, we are giddy about a single access point for all of our online business transactions, not to mention online scheduling on the horizon.

I've always said, once we master access, no one, I mean NO ONE, will be able to hold a candle to us. Watch out competitors, here we come!

So consider this Epic moment a fresh beginning, and imagine the places we can go from here.

Thank you for all you do,
Amy

⊙ REFLECTION

Ah, Epic. This was an unexpected but much-needed technological improvement and investment for our system. I remember when it was announced. We'd embark on a process lasting 18 to 24 months to implement Epic—a new EMR (electronic medical record) system for Emory Healthcare. For those that know about technology transitions, this was a big one. And those months truly whizzed by.

My favorite comment from an advertising rep was about Epic. She reached out to me via email to reconnect. I said I was happy to but we had our Epic go-live ahead of us and I couldn't spare the time then. When we finally had lunch, she told me she thought Epic go-live meant we were getting ready to launch an amazing new advertising campaign! Proof positive that our health care lingo does not resonate outside our internal teams.

Subject: Making wishes reality

Date: Friday, October 14, 2022, 5:06 p.m.

Team,

French pilot and author of *Le Petit Prince*, Antoine de Saint-Exupery[47] once said, ***"A goal without a plan is just a wish."***

Another iteration of our FY23 mantra — *"Stop Talking, Start Doing"* — but with a twist. The plan is critical. Otherwise you are doing for doing's sake, but not working toward any achievable goal.

Epic, once a wish of many of our providers, became reality when Emory Healthcare identified Epic as a realistic goal and developed a plan, using a series of SMART goals[48] and mini-plans (or sprints), to bring that goal to life.

Our October 1 go-live is a wish more than a decade in the making, with the goal formulation and plan taking three years to accomplish.

Three years, you say? Yes, at least three years.

The implementation plan to go-live was a 24-month plan. However, at least a year, if not two or more, preceded the announcement in 2020 of our move to Epic. Months of cost-benefit analysis, scenario planning, visits to Epic-based health care systems, and contract negotiations.

Likewise our CRM journey took nearly seven years to materialize, and also more than a decade as a wish. Fortunately, that wish turned into a realistic goal. We added a detailed plan (and a few curveballs along the way) and that wish, too, became reality.

This team, each of you, mission critical in making both of those wishes come true.

As I mentioned in Huddle this morning, our FY23 planning is not yet complete. It is now time to solidify our SMART goals and develop an action plan (including scheduled tactics, deadlines, milestones and deployments) to bring our FY23 wishes to life.

Marketing in FY23 is different. Much more focused on patient and customer communications. It is highly targeted to retain and engage with our existing customers and active leads. We aim to develop a relationship with our patients and potential customers in order to drive loyalty and move them through the funnel to conversion. This is the new age for health care marketing. And as Denise reported, Salesforce says Emory Healthcare is leading the industry in this manner.

So here's to the trailblazers—YOU. How will you bring your wishes to life with goals and an action plan?

I can't wait to see the paths you lay ahead for us and look back at the end of FY23 on the amazing wishes you made come true.

Thank you for all you do,
Amy

Subject: Maleficent Returns

Date: Friday, October 28, 2022, 8:42 p.m.

Team,

A late edition Friday email...

No rain and no appendix this year = no stopping Maleficent power-walking her way to a personal best at tonight's Monster Dash 5k. The annual race benefits Josh's high school: Rockdale Magnet School for Science and Technology.

How will you spend your Halloween weekend?

Spookily yours,

Maleficent

 REFLECTION

Finally, I got to participate in my first Monster Dash to support Josh's Magnet school. It didn't happen his freshman year because of the pandemic. His sophomore year's race got canceled for rain, and two days later my appendix wanted out. So this was the reprise.

I clocked my fastest walking 5K I could remember—in full costume! I wasn't quite sure if my child was proud or embarrassed by me, probably a little bit of both, but since he was the one who suggested I go as Maleficent the first time—*and* was my costume consultant—I had to do it.

The cheers from the students and the teachers at the checkpoints gave me great joy, bringing out my inner kid and my inner competition. Never having done this course before, I loved experiencing every turn and vista. My favorite part, especially in my costume, was race-walking through the cemetery. Well, that and power walking past some other parents. I may not be a runner like the front of the line, but I was determined to finish as fast as my walking legs would take me past my middle-aged peers.

The course ends on the race track surrounding the football and soccer field. It was my first time being on the pitch where I watched Josh play on the varsity soccer team. Catching my breath and cooling down, I soaked it all in.

Alas, there were no costume contests to win. But if there were, I surely would have. As I'd learn a year later, apparently, I'm the only mom to go all out in costume for this thing. I really thought I'd win my age group, but I didn't. Other parents with still-working knees and who actually enjoy running won.

Fast forward a year later to October 2023. And, I have a theory. I was 50 for that 2022 race. Most of Josh's friends' parents are younger than me and Chris, by several years if not a decade plus. It's entirely possible I fell into the 35 to 50 age group. If that is the case, there's no chance I'd win.

A year later, at age 51, I found myself nearly 10 pounds heavier due to two months of sinus infections and burgeoning perimenopause (not for the faint of heart!). But I still walked and dressed out—this time as Wonder Woman.

I walked my heart out, ending with my worst 5K time in my walking history memory. Hubs and son had other commitments that night, so I stayed for the awards anyway to see if I might win a raffle prize. Well, what to my wondering ears should I hear? Amy Comeau—first place in the final age group! They didn't say the age range, but at 51 apparently I beat out a bunch of parents and grandparents who either had stroller duty or were happy walking at a leisurely pace.

I was the last medal given. They were clearly tired of taking photos, but I walked right over to have mine taken! I was unexpectedly proud. Thrilled! Humbled and feeling slightly ridiculous. So I took myself out to dinner afterwards to celebrate the win.

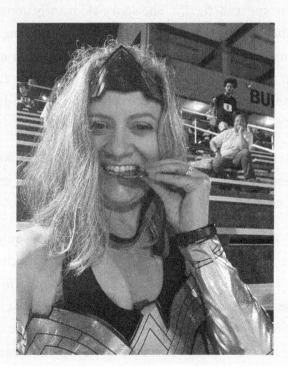

✉ **Subject: The Tale of Two Wolves**

Date: Friday, December 16, 2022, 5:13 p.m.

Team,

This week I had the good fortune to attend Winship's Town Hall and Holiday Party in person. Jenny and her team put on an incredible event highlighting the amazing and important work our Winship teams do to improve lives and provide hope by lessening the burden of cancer in our communities. And I got to see and hug friends and colleagues across Emory, and some I literally haven't seen IRL in years.

Part of the town hall included a reflection from Winship's director of spiritual health. She spoke eloquently about the role all members of the team play in cancer care, making a special point to mention non-clinical-care-delivery roles such as food and nutrition, environmental services, valet, call center agents and more. It takes a team to deliver the care and make the discoveries that make Winship a world-class cancer program.

Caroline closed with the "Tale of Two Wolves," a Cherokee parable about good and evil. It is one I hadn't heard previously and I found it profound. It goes like this:

> **THE TWO WOLVES A CHEROKEE STORY** A young boy came to his Grandfather, filled with anger at another boy who had done him an injustice. The old Grandfather said to his grandson, "Let me tell you a story. I too, at times, have felt a great hate for those that have taken so much, with no sorrow for what they do. But hate wears you down, and hate does not hurt your enemy. Hate is like

taking poison and wishing your enemy would die. I have struggled with these feelings many times."

"It is as if there are two wolves inside me; one wolf is good and does no harm. He lives in harmony with all around him and does not take offence when no offence was intended. He will only fight when it is right to do so, and in the right way. But the other wolf, is full of anger. The littlest thing will set him into a fit of temper. He fights everyone, all the time, for no reason. He cannot think because his anger and hate are so great. It is helpless anger, because his anger will change nothing. Sometimes it is hard to live with these two wolves inside me, because both of the wolves try to dominate my spirit."

The boy looked into his Grandfather's eyes. "Which wolf will win, Grandfather?" The Grandfather smiled and said, "The one I feed."

And the very next day, a friend posted this quote on her social channels, reinforcing the lesson in the Cherokee parable.

"Becoming less reactive is a huge part of growth and decreasing stress. If you let everything get you worked up, you're damaging your mind, body and spirit."—@slimarela_

Some have called me overly optimistic or Pollyanna. Perhaps I am, or it's the meditation[49] influence talking, but I instinctively have chosen to fuel the good. That doesn't mean the evil wolf doesn't pop out from time to time, but that's when I apply @_slimarela's approach to tame it. As I've focused on this, I have found myself more grounded and better able to navigate life's complexities.

How about you? Which wolf do you choose to feed?

Thank you for all you do,
Amy

2023

✉ Subject: Cardiac Feelings

Date: Friday, January 6, 2023, 5:22 p.m.

Team,

When you are born in Buffalo, you are born a Buffalo Bills fan. It's part of your DNA.

We love our team, and we are proud people who defend our city as it often gets made fun of for our snow, nasal accents, and crazy table-crashing fans. In fact, when I was growing up one of our city's slogans was: Buffalo, We're Talking Proud! For those of you following the Damar Hamlin story, you're getting a glimpse into the heart of our town, the City of Good Neighbors.

You can imagine my distress watching Damar Hamlin collapse on Monday Night Football. I shared with some of you that I really could not sleep that night, not knowing if he was alive or dead. This has been a roller-coaster week of emotions—with the thrilling news today that he is off the ventilator, Facetimed his teammates and appears to have full neurological function.

I'm sharing this, however, not only because it's important to me personally. **It's important to us professionally**.

This easily could have happened at a home Falcons game, even a Hawks, Braves, or Dream game. In that scenario, our Emory Healthcare providers would be on the field and among the first responders: Dr. Jonathan Kim[50], our sports cardiologist; Dr. David Wright, or a member of his emergency medicine team; Dr. Kyle Hammond[51] and our sports medicine team, and our Emory School of Medicine at Grady colleagues.

And it happens to people every day, most of whom do not receive media attention nor benefit from the swift medical attention as Damar. Sadly, nearly 400,000 people die from sudden cardiac arrest annually in the United States.

It brings our mantra of Improving Lives and Providing Hope into clear view. Our providers and researchers are working every day to find new and better ways to diagnose, prevent and treat heart problems, including cardiac arrest. It makes our work in educating our communities on the warning signs of heart attack and the importance of CPR and AEDs, as well as marketing our heart and vascular program evermore real and meaningful.

Thank you for allowing me space to talk about it this week and, if you have made it this far, thank you for reading.

As always thank you for all you do.

Go Bills!
Amy

P.S. If you are like me and thought cardiac arrest and heart attack were synonymous—they are not. The AHA has a very good description of the differences[52], including that a heart attack can result in cardiac arrest, which contributes to the mistaken synonym assumption.

⬤ REFLECTION

We all know now that Damar Hamlin has made a full and complete recovery from his cardiac arrest, crediting University of Cincinnati and Buffalo physicians for his recovery.

Bills trainer Denny Kellington delivered the life-saving CPR, earning his own 15 minutes of fame. He and the Bills' training staff and physicians earned an ESPY and were recognized with the Pat Tillman Award for Service. At the July 2023 event, Bills' head trainer Nate Breske spoke on the importance of funding for CPR training and AEDs (Automatic External Defibrillators).[53]

"This story is about a lot of things, but to us it's about raising awareness of cardiac events, which happen every day, in so many different places. Please, support funding for AED and CPR training, especially in underserved communities. As well as the need for athletic trainers in youth sports. If there's one thing you take away from this tonight: Learn CPR and how to use an AED, because they save lives. Set a goal for yourself. Do it this summer before football season. You don't have to be perfect. We always say, "doing something is better than doing nothing.""

Hamlin was back on the team and played five games in the 2023 season. In early November 2023, the Bills and Bengals rematched for Sunday Night Football. Hamlin was not active for the game. Although the Bills lost the game, they won in my book because Hamlin is alive and healthy. He celebrated his recovery by having dinner with his entire University of Cincinnati Health care team and funded 10 scholarships in their names.[54]

✉ Subject: The Fosbury Flop

Date: Friday, January 20, 2023, 5:00 p.m.

Team,

This morning I had the pleasure of hearing Rohit Bhargava[55] talk about "Non-Obvious Trends That Matter For Your Industry." He's made his career trying to spot the unusual. In essence, finding ways to innovate.

He opened with a story about the Fosbury Flop.[56]

Raise of hands: how many of you actually know about the Fosbury Flop?

I had heard of it, but honestly couldn't remember the story, until Rohit went on to describe it.

Dick Fosbury won Olympic gold for the high jump in 1968, the only competitor to go over the bar "back first." Can you imagine, competing at the Olympics and here comes this guy jumping completely the opposite of what you've learned and not only winning, but setting an Olympic world record? Now 75, Fosbury revolutionized the sport and today no one competes in high jump the old way.

Fosbury developed a non-obvious, but better, way to compete. That's innovation.

Rohit, who is also an Emory University alum[57], spent the rest of the time sharing some non-obvious trends[58] and teaching us his Haystack Method[59] of finding them. Hint: it uses a lot of Post-it notes!

He challenged us all as marketers to practice non-obvious thinking, saying "If you do that, you can anticipate the future and help direct your company."

I know we often feel that pointing out the OBVIOUS to our company is revolutionary. Think patient retention campaigns or fully loaded physician profiles delivering better results. But imagine if we pair that with NON-OBVIOUS thinking?

(Or perhaps our patient retention campaign IS an example of non-obvious thinking? I know we hear from colleagues across the country how ground-breaking that work is in health care.)

I'd love to hear what are some non-obvious trends you are seeing? Or how will you apply non-obvious thinking to your work?

Thank you for all you do,
Amy

Every Storm Runs Out of Rain

✉️ **Subject: People who understand people**

Date: Friday, January 27, 2023, 4:56 p.m.

Team,

At last night's Marketing Executive Advisory Committee (MEAC), I shared the quote: **"The people who understand people always win."** Another gem from Rohit Bhargava of the Non-Obvious Company.

Again, an obvious statement that masquerades as non-obvious, especially when it is easy for Emory to fall into the groupthink of navel-gazing.

Our role as marketers is to serve as the Voice of the Customer[60]. Those of you who participated in the focus groups or last night's MEAC saw the power of our patients' and potential patients' voices firsthand. In the course of six months, we went from an over-engineered, inward-facing academic brand positioning statement to one that evokes humanity and appeals to our customers and employees, while remaining uniquely Emory Healthcare.

Never forget the power of the Voice of the Customer, as our patients are whom we serve and why Emory Healthcare exists. Through our patient and family-centered care model[61], we promise to Improve Lives and Provide Hope.

Thank you for all you do each and every day to bring our care model and that promise to the communities we serve.

Thank you,
Amy

PRO TIP

When you are having challenges getting your internal stakeholders and leaders to understand and truly hear the *why* from your customers, show them. Literally.

We spent 18 months working on updating our brand positioning statement alongside the creation of our employee value proposition. This took a lot of work. Our marketing and recruitment agencies partnered together. We analyzed first- and third-party research, including an ethnographic listening study. We surveyed our employees and held 10 internal focus groups. From there we met with nearly 20 internal stakeholder and patient advisor groups to get their feedback on the proposed statement.

Even still, when we got to our executive team and physician-leader groups, they insisted on including "eminent" in the statement. We told them that made us look arrogant and inaccessible to our customers. Already battling a perceived accessibility issue, this would only reinforce that. So, we tested it. We already had focus groups planned to get feedback on creative concepts, so we added the brand positioning to the discussion guide.

And boy, did it work! All three of the focus groups reacted negatively to the word. Saying it made the health system look arrogant. When asked what system they thought it was, one person said: "That's GOTTA be Emory. Only Emory would say they are eminent."

I had our agency create a 12-minute video of clips from those focus groups and shared it with our executive team. I told them it may feel awkward to watch a 12-minute video during our meeting, but it was important for them to hear our patients, and patients of our competitors, talk about us in their own words. Far more powerful than reading their quotes in a paper report. It worked. We eliminated "eminent" from our lexicon and landed on a brand positioning that is true to Emory Healthcare and resonates with our audiences.

Subject: Upside Down

Date: Friday, February 3, 2023, 4:59 p.m.

Team,

Today's upside down and sideways Zoom capers got me thinking about *Where the Sidewalk Ends*, by Shel Silverstein[62].

That and his *A Light in the Attic*[63] book were staples in my house growing up. Well-worn and dog-eared, my sisters and I fought over them.

In fact, I still remember reciting "Sarah Silvia Cynthia Stout Would Not Take the Garbage Out" in eighth grade English class during our poetry segment. I'll never forget Mr. Elston, smiling, shaking his head at me and telling me to *slow down*. I was nervous and wanted to get it over with as fast as possible. No matter how many times I tried to slow down, I just couldn't. Even "slow me" was fast.

After this morning's antics, I recalled Shel Silverstein had a poem about being "upside-down".

I don't have the Moudy Family edition of the books, and I'm not sure where they are. Did one of my sisters end up with them or are they on a shelf at my parents' house in Buffalo? Hm. . . Anyway, I went to trusty Google to see what I could find.

After a bit of Googling, I found it! The poem is called **"Reflection."**[64] How many of you are familiar with Shel Silverstein and what's your favorite poem of his? If not, be sure to check him out— delightful and accessible poetry for kids and adults!

I'm thankful our upside-down Zoom prompted this walk down memory lane. Hope this brings a smile to your face as it does mine.

Have a terrific weekend,
Amy

> 💬 **REFLECTION**
>
> Zoom was having issues that day where several of my team's individual video boxes displayed sideways or upside down and kept changing throughout the meeting. It reminded of Shel Sliverstein's poem "Upside Down." In a few short lines, he perfectly captures how to see things from someone else's point of view. In it, he describes a man looking at his reflection in a puddle calling him "Upside-Down Man" and ending "Maybe he is right side up and I am upside down."

Subject: The Wise Heart

Date: Friday, February 10, 2023, 5:55 p.m.

Team,

It's been a heavy week with the catastrophic earthquake in Turkey and Syria (its death toll sadly still rising) and closer to home the news of our needed financial mitigation to help guide us through industry disruption. I'm feeling it and I'm sure you are too.

I was going to lighten things up by talking about the Super Bowl or sharing my Chia pet experiment, but that seemed almost too light. Maybe next week instead. . .

Then I read the story in today's Emory Report about "One Emory"[65], where guidance from the Dalai Lama[66] grounded me. Reminding me of not only Emory Healthcare's core purpose, but EMORY's purpose. I'll share it here:

> *Emory's mission is "to create, preserve, teach, and apply knowledge in the service of humanity." The motto is, "The wise heart seeks knowledge." Both the mission and motto refer to knowledge and the fact that having and sharing knowledge confers great responsibility. In India, President Gregory Fenves says the Dalai Lama, who is Presidential Distinguished Professor at Emory, reminded him that there must be heart in the classroom. "His Holiness radiates peace and his message to our small group was about compassion — that compassion must be a fundamental part of education if we are to heal the world," Fenves said.*

Heart. Knowledge. Compassion. Wisdom. In the service of humanity.

Yessss. This. This is who we are. Why we exist.

Why EMORY—both Healthcare and University—are driven and called to serve.

So, on those tough days, those down days, have compassion for yourself and for others. For it's through our hearts and our heads that we will improve lives and provide hope, not only for humanity, but also for ourselves.

Thank you for all you do,
Amy

✉@ **Subject: Sophia Chia**

Date: Friday, February 17, 2023, 5:41 p.m.

Team,

As foreshadowed last week, I am definitely lightening things up with this Friday's email. And by special request from Lindsay, who expressed interest in my Chia Pet experiment.

First, let's ground ourselves in the Chia Pet history.

The Chia Pet[67], with its zippy jingle, transcends all generations. It debuted in 1977, gained fame in the 1980s, and by 2019 has sold 15 million units worldwide.

Today Chia features many different brand extensions and licensing deals. Hence, my Golden Girls chia pet. But wait, there's more! Bob Ross, Mandalorian, Star Wars, Willie Nelson, Minions, and even horror characters like Chucky and Michael Meyers.

One Christmas during the pandemic (not sure which, they all run together), my husband got me a Sophia Chia pet as an impulse buy. I came across it two weekends ago while cleaning up the house and decided to give it a whirl.

Bottom Line: It's messy and not at all what the ads portray. FALSE ADVERTISING!

She's been planted for the suggested 14 days now. Instead of a lovely and full houseplant, Sophia has a weird Chia mullet and alopecia. Mold on top, crazy chia sprout party in the back, bald spots throughout.

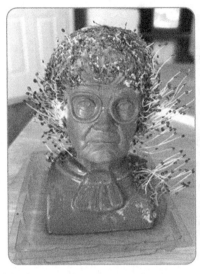 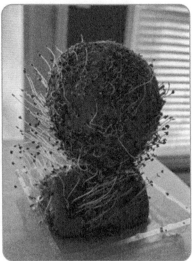

Not sure what happened: is it the shape of her head (smaller surface area than the OG chia pets)? Were my chia seeds too old? Did I make the paste too thin? Who knows. Regardless, it has been an amusing experiment.

So, there you have it, my first ever Chia pet experiment. Bonus: I can wipe the Chia mullet off and try her again and again.

Here's hoping your weekend fares better than Sophia Chia. Unless a moldy Chia mullet party is your style. In which case, party on!

Thanks for all you do,
Amy

✉ Subject: You are Lifesavers

Date: Friday, March 3, 2023, 5:05 p.m.

Team,

Those of you on Huddle this morning heard me share kudos from Emory Healthcare Network (EHN) leadership for our efforts. For this week's Friday send-off email, I'd like to further connect the dots.

EHN's new Chief Quality and Medical Officer, asked me to emphasize with you that our work helps improve quality outcomes for our patients and thus both improving and proving Emory Healthcare's quality care. Here's a quick look at that coming to life:

- One in eight women[68] will be diagnosed with breast cancer in her/their lifetime.*
- Early diagnosis leads to better outcomes.
- When found early, breast cancer is one of the most curable cancers.
  - » *MedicalNewsToday*[69] lists breast cancer as its number one curable cancer when found early.
  - » According to the National Breast Cancer Foundation[70]: "When breast cancer is detected early, and is in the localized stage, the five-year relative survival rate is 99%"

Our most recent email campaign promoting mammography led to 665 calls for appointment. For the sake of argument, let's assume all schedule and get their screening mammogram.

- 10% of screening mammograms are abnormal, but most are false positives[71].

- According to MedicineNet[72]: "Of all women who get regular mammograms, only about 5% will be found to have breast cancer."

- Assuming all 665 callers get screened, one-half percent of them will be diagnosed with breast cancer. That's four individuals (technically 3.24, but you cannot have ¼ of a person, so I rounded up).

Because of the work you do, 665 of our patients made the call to get screened. In this scenario, **you've been the catalyst to find four cancers early, allowing four women and non-binary individuals assigned female at birth the best chance of survival**. And if they choose Winship for their care, their chances of survival are 25% higher[73] than those who choose non-NCI-designated cancer centers.

Don't ever think for a minute that the work you do is not important. It is. It is literally lifesaving.

While this may be a breast-cancer example, it translates easily to nearly every service line and all the work we do. Each and every one of you has a role in Improving Lives and Providing Hope.

So, remember this: **You are patient facing. You are saving lives. You are essential health care workers.**

Thank you for all you do,
Amy

PRO TIP

NCI is the acronym for National Cancer Institute[74], from whom cancer centers across the country can apply for a rigorous grant that earns them NCI designation, either as a National Cancer Institute-designated center or a National Cancer Institute-designated comprehensive cancer center.

✉@ **Subject: Ode to Beatriz**

Date: Friday, March 10, 2023, 4:37 p.m.

Team,

Earlier this week on LinkedIn, I shared a personal tribute to a woman who had a big impact on my life early in my career: Beatriz Iorgulescu. I'd like to share it with you here, so you can learn a little bit more about her, but also take a moment to reflect on those people who have had a lasting impact on your own life or career.

While Beatriz and I only worked together for two years, she has made a lasting impression on me.

We lost touch over the years, but the advent of social media allowed us to reconnect about a decade ago. We exchange holiday cards and Facebook messages from time to time, and always talk about trying to meet up whenever I'm in Chicago. I think of her often and reflect on how powerful and formative those two years at Lyric Opera of Chicago were for my career, shaping my work ethic and soaking up marketing, communications, and fundraising best practices.

Is there anyone like Beatriz who has made a similar impact on your life? If so, I'd love to learn more about them and how they impacted your career.

Thank you for all you do; and my everlasting thanks to Beatriz,

Amy

◯ REFLECTION

I could literally write a book on my career path—from getting into Northwestern as a voice major, realizing how hard it would be to literally sing for my supper, minoring in Music Business, multiple internships, and my first real job as an administrative assistant at Lyric Opera of Chicago. How did I go from the performing arts to health care? Well, that's a whole story and you'll need to wait to read the book when I write it.

At Lyric, I supported one of their five fundraising boards: Chapters, like regional fan clubs or opera guilds, nearly 35 of them across Chicagoland. Beatriz was on the Chapters Board, so I spent a lot of time with her. An immigrant, English was her second language, so she always asked me for help with her English. In turn, whether she knew it or not, she became a mentor to me. My second female mentor in my young career (the first was Melissa Sharp Leasia, my supervisor when I interned my junior year of college with the Chicago Children's Choir).

Beatriz became my mom away from home. When it came time for our first and only Henri Bendel Fashion Show fundraiser, she got me one of her rooms at the Union Club of Chicago (where the event was held), so I did not have to travel home to my Evanston studio apartment at midnight. I still remember having breakfast with her the next morning, just the two of us.

My mom was especially thankful to have Beatriz looking after me. And I'm thrilled I got the chance for the two of them to meet. One summer, when my mom came to visit me (probably to hear me perform with the Grant Park Music Festival choir), the Chapters' board had a small Bastille Day picnic luncheon. My mom is a retired French teacher, so this was right up her alley.

Fast forward to June 2023 when I attended my first performance at Lyric Opera of Chicago in 30 years, splurging on a Box seat for *West Side Story*. I was completely unprepared for my overwhelming emotional response walking into the lobby. So many hours spent there over 30 years ago, making $17,000 annually and checking in important donors for events like the Opera Ball or working open dress rehearsals.

I saw my first Ring Cycle at Lyric. Heard amazing artists like Sam Ramey, Jane Eaglen, Bryn Terfel, Renee Fleming and Kiri Te Kanawa... It was only two years, but it is burned into my memory, far stronger than places where I've worked longer. So many experiences, so much learned.

I realize now how much those two years shaped my philosophy on marketing for what I learned as obvious from 1994-96, like monthly annual fund renewals, a DOS (disc-operating system)-based but super effective CRM system, and even the debut of Microsoft Office. Remember Clippy? Yes, this all dates me, but I wouldn't trade my experience at Lyric for the world. It is the foundation of my career.

✉@ **Subject: I wish we had started at Emory**

Date: Friday, March 24, 2023, 3:37 p.m.

"I wish we had started at Emory. . .but now it's too late."

Team,

This is a quote I heard today from a woman whose husband has stage 4 brain cancer, a glioblastoma[75].

I heard a very similar quote, earlier this year, from a longtime colleague of mine whose husband had emergency surgery at a competitor to remove a football-sized tumor from his abdomen, known as a GIST[76], a rare GI cancer.

Their words haunt me.

"I wish we had started at Emory. . ."

Both were diagnosed in August. The former is "not on hospice yet," getting treatment out of state. I helped the latter seek a second opinion from Dr. Ken Cardona[77], our GIST specialist. And they are not the first people I've heard say these words.

". . .but now it's too late."

On the cusp of our Winship at Emory Midtown TV ad shoot next week, hearing these words today immediately and emotionally re-grounded me on why health care marketing matters. Why marketing EMORY HEALTHCARE matters.

Where you go first matters—The very 'reason to believe' anchoring our upcoming Orthopaedics & Spine, Winship, and Heart & Vascular campaigns. But people don't know to come to

Emory unless we (yes, we) persuade them. Your work matters. Your work—informing, educating, engaging, and helping people find and choose Emory for their health care—absolutely matters.

It makes all the difference between: *"Emory saved my life!"* and *"I wish we had started at Emory. . ."* Quite literally the difference between life and death.

So, let's do all we can to eliminate the words *"I wish we had started at Emory. . .but now it's too late"* from people's mouths. And let's recommit together to doing all we can to continue to **Improve Lives and Provide Hope**.

Thank you for all you do,
Amy

✉ Subject: There are no losses

Date: Friday, April 28, 2023, 5:10 p.m.

Team,

We've spoken of it much this week, but Jenny, the Winship team and all of you who volunteered executed an amazing NACCDO-PAMN (National Association of Cancer Center Development Officers and Public Affairs and Marketing Network) conference. Together you showed the entire NCI cancer center universe just how amazing Emory, Winship, and Atlanta are.

As a volunteer, I got to sit in on many great sessions and plenary talks. Influencer Nicole Walters[78] opened the conference sharing a personal story[79] of how her daughter was diagnosed with and now survived stage 4 Hodgkin's lymphoma—thanks to the great care at Winship.

Our own Laura kept a standing-room-only crowd rapt giving insights on how to develop great content with a small team. Many praised the collaborative relationship between the health system and the NCI cancer center. And Jenny, alongside peers from Penn Medicine and University of Miami, shared trade secrets on how to build influence with your leadership team to get the resources you need.

Then, yesterday, the conference closed out with Monica Pearson interviewing former Atlanta Falcons' quarterback Matt Ryan. As you know, we have a direct partnership with Matt Ryan for marketing. When he was traded to the Colts, we chose to maintain the relationship but direct it in support of Winship at Emory Midtown this year. Many thanks to Larry for helping with Matt's involvement at the conference and next week's ribbon cutting.

Monica, a masterful interviewer, got Matt to open up about playing in the NFL, his trade to Indy, his nickname "Matty Ice," facing adversity, who non-football Matt is, tips for fundraisers and communicators making asks, and finally on leadership.

Matt shared some incredible insights from coaches and mentors in his life. The one that resonated with me the most is this from his high school coach and math teacher:

"There are no losses. You either win or you learn. That's what the L is for."

What a profound and meaningful statement. One that can be applied far beyond sports. So, the next time you feel you lost at something, instead of ruminating in the loss, ponder the learning. What did you learn from that experience and what will you do differently next time?

Thank you for all you do,
Amy

◯ REFLECTION

This was a super busy time for me. In a span of eight weeks I had a Vizient Chief Marketing and Strategy Officers Meeting in Dallas, my boss's sudden departure, our Winship TV shoot, our son's spring break, Easter, speaking at the HMPS (Healthcare Marketing and Physician Strategies) Forum, hosting NACCDO-PAMN in Atlanta, followed by our Winship Emory Midtown opening.

On top of all of that, I suffered from a right ear infection that I must have picked up over spring break. It peaked over Easter weekend and fortunately I got antibiotics from urgent care before the HMPS Forum. Even still, I was slightly deaf that whole week and remember laboring through both my presentation and a podcast I recorded. Just as it felt like it was clearing, it decided to shift to a left sinus infection as I moved into our NACCDO-PAMN conference and Winship opening. I was sick for six weeks straight—it was rough.

Between the sickness and the uncertainty at work with the beginning of a litany of leadership changes, I found Matt Ryan's life lessons comforting.

"What matters is your ability to adjust, adapt and react."—Yes.

"It's important to be flexible. Know who you are leading. But know your non-negotiables too."—Yes.

"It doesn't get easier. The folks who are successful are the ones who can handle the hard. Face and deal with the adversity. Life doesn't get easier. It's hard."—Also, yes.

And then he said this as he contemplated his next professional move, knowing, but unable to say his playing days were over because of contractual obligations: "The next step is just that. The next step. Not the final step."

His words spoke volumes to me. Still do.

✉ **Subject: Mercury in Retrograde**

Date: Friday, May 5, 2023, 6:15 p.m.

Team,

I intended to write today's Friday email to cap off a fabulous week of Winship at Emory Midtown openings and excitement around our campaigns launching **next week!!**

Then, we had the active shooter tragedy on Wednesday that cast a pall over the celebrations and reminded us ever-so-close-to-home why we do the active shooter trainings every year. As I read more news reports recounting the situation, I'm further disturbed and saddened by how the health care system failed this gentleman who both served our country and suffers from mental illness. Another reminder of the important and healing work of our Emory Healthcare Veterans Program. I'm finding the words to describe and reflect on this difficult.

Instead, I thought I'd bring you all in on the astrological phenomenon of "Mercury in Retrograde."[80] Yes, it could be considered hogwash, but once I learned what it was, I've noticed its impact nearly every single time.

This article[81] from *The Atlantic* does a good job explaining Mercury in Retrograde, but essentially this is a time when Mercury orbits the Sun slower than the Earth. Usually, Mercury orbits the Sun faster than us. Astrologists believe the activity of the planets has an impact on us as humans. During times of retrograde, things go wonky.

The Today Show[82] describes it this way: *"Mercury rules communication, travel, news, information, gossip and technology. This means that we can expect meltdowns, false gossip, miscommunications, technology fails (which is why it's best to back up files and contacts before the retrograde), issues in travel, missed connections and delays in hearing pertinent information."*

Sound familiar? The transplant/vaccine social media flare-up last week. Our Google payment issues this week. Heck, even the Writers Guild strike.

We are smackdab in the middle of retrograde: April 21 through May 14. We've got one week to go. . .so hang on to your hats.

I became familiar with Mercury in Retrograde more than two decades ago when I bought my condo. My first time as a homeowner. A colleague of mine at the Atlanta Opera urged me not to close on my condo during Mercury in Retrograde. I thought he was just superstitious and ignored him.

I shouldn't have.

While I adored my condo, I ended up selling it for a loss in 2004. And while living there, I suffered through the ice maker in my refrigerator flooding my kitchen and ruining my hardwood floors. Not once, but twice!

I have been a believer ever since.

But Mercury in Retrograde is not always a bad thing[83]. It teaches us to slow down, be contemplative. So, while technology and communications go haywire, think of it as the planets telling us to chill out for a minute.

I'm not asking you to subscribe to the Mercury in Retrograde theory, but now you know what we're talking about when we throw out the *"Oh, it must be Mercury in Retrograde"* references.

In the spirit of the good side of retrograde, I encourage you all to take this weekend to *slow down*, rest, and find time for yourselves. Mother Earth and Mercury prescribe it.

If you've made it this far, thanks for humoring me. And if you're a convert like me, I would love to hear your Mercury in Retrograde story.

Thank you for all you do,
Amy

✉ Subject: Anticlimactic

Date: Friday, May 12, 2023, 5:02 p.m.

Team,

Take a moment and remember where you were on March 11, 2020. The day the World Health Organization (WHO) declared COVID-19 a global pandemic[84].

Do you remember the fear and uncertainty you felt? That we all felt?

Shortly thereafter we were sent home to "shelter in place" for the next eight weeks, naively thinking that doing so would allow COVID-19 to pass right by us and fizzle out. How wrong we were.

In the three years since, MILLIONS of people have died from COVID-19. More than 6.9 million people[85] at the latest count according to the WHO—that's equivalent to the entire population of the state of Indiana! And more than 785 million reported cases—which we know must soar far beyond one billion given how many cases are no longer reported. (Makes McDonald's "more than one billion served" tag line pale in comparison.)

Yesterday, the U.S. Department of Health and Human Services declared the end of the COVID-19 Public Health Emergency[86].

Seems pretty anticlimactic, doesn't it?

Where's the fanfare? The trumpets, the cheers, the celebration? Something that literally changed our lives and how we live and work forever should not end with a whisper, when it came in with a roar.

I think back on these Friday emails and remember how hopeless and dark some weeks felt. The unknown, the mental toll, the grief of what once was that is no longer. I sometimes found it hard to find the words to inspire. But each week I found hope somewhere, a tiny glimpse of the light at the end of the very long tunnel.

While many would like to quickly throw the pandemic in the trash and forget about it. I never want to forget.

It was a remarkable time to work in health care.

We felt every single moment of the pandemic. We were fortunate to be at the source of science and truth, more so than anyone else. Emory Healthcare with the highest COVID-19 survival rates[87] not just in the nation, but the world. Our Emory scientists and researchers advanced science, bringing the Moderna vaccine[88] and Molnupiravir[89] antiviral treatment to the world. Literally Improving Lives and Providing Hope.

A truly global historic moment in time. That all of us are fortunate to have survived. Our children's children won't believe it when they're told the stories of 2020 and 2021. What will the history books say about these years?

So no, it should not go out with a whisper. It should not be forgotten. Too many people died, too many people's families changed forever. Moms not here to be celebrated this Mother's Day weekend, nor children here to celebrate their mothers. People still dying daily from COVID-19[90] (April 2023 averaged six COVID-19 deaths per day in Georgia). **No, we cannot forget.**

For those of you who have been part of this team from the very beginning of the pandemic, you know exactly what I mean. For those of you who joined us recently or somewhere in between, I'm sure you too are experiencing what it means to work in health care and especially at Emory. We're privileged every day to advance science, inspire hope, and help our communities get the care they need to live a rich and fulfilling life.

At the end of Health Care Week, I thank each and every one of you for being part of our team. And for the roles you have played in helping the pandemic be a thing of the past. Something to remember, learn from and grow.

This weekend take a quiet moment for your own reflection on the past three years and then raise a glass of your favorite beverage to toast the end of the COVID-19 public emergency. We really are on the other side of it now.

Thank you for all you do,
Amy

Epilogue

"One day this is going to be over—can you imagine that day? How we'll come out into the sun and laugh and hug and sing and dance and hold hands? I'm living for that day. It'll be like nothing we've experienced before."—Glennon Doyle, *One Day This Is Going to Be Over*

We know now that Glennon Doyle was wrong.

While the height of the pandemic is behind us, coronavirus is still alive and well in our world. In fact, we're seeing news reports[91] of a surge of COVID-19 cases this summer of 2024.

I, myself, have now had COVID twice: once in June 2022 and again this past January 2024.

We never hit herd immunity, but the virus has weakened significantly as vaccines and our own immune systems help fight it. It's just a part of our daily lives now, like the common cold or the flu.

All thanks to modern medicine, science and the people who made this happen—from scientists to manufacturers to pharmacists to truck drivers, and yes, marketers and communicators.

As life got back to normal and the pandemic ended with a whimper, people forgot about COVID-19, no longer the deadly threat to our world's existence.

So, no, we never did get our day to "come out into the sun and laugh and hug and sing and dance and hold hands" like Glennon predicted.

We have, however, made it through, finally getting to the other side of the very long tunnel – now laughing, hugging, singing and dancing with our friends and families just as if the pandemic never happened.

That is a good and glorious thing.

But let us never forget the impact the pandemic had on our world, our society, our workplaces, our economies and our people. Some good, some not-so-good.

We must remember and mourn the millions of lives lost.

In remembering and reflecting, we honor their lives. We also bring ourselves the closure we need to put the pandemic behind us—a chapter left for the history books.

Now that you have finished this book, please take a quiet moment to reflect on how the pandemic impacted you and raise a glass of your favorite beverage to toast a new beginning.

Thank you for reading my story,

Amy

Appendix

1   https://www.latimes.com/science/story/2020-04-08/la-sci-pandemic-fighting-doctor
2   https://hbr.org/2020/03/that-discomfort-youre-feeling-is-grief
3   Double Chocolate Brownies, p. 287, Martha Stewart's COOKIES, 2008, by Martha Stewart Living Omnimedia, Inc., Clarkson Potter/Publishers, an imprint of the Crown Publishing Group, a division of Random House, Inc., New York.
4   https://open.spotify.com/show/5S8mLIy88umlW6I2zjST5J?si=26278060abdb4df1
5   https://open.spotify.com/show/0dfJjJyNxF9iW7zmBtLnBf?si=ae47e2b85d2a4255
6   https://www.youtube.com/watch?v=jOu7fzj0AiA&ab_channel=GeorgiaHospitalAssociation
7   https://www.amazon.com/10-Happier-Self-Help-Actually-Works/dp/0062265431
8   https://www.amazon.com/Essentials-Health-Care-Marketing-Berkowitz/dp/1284200159
9   https://www.youtube.com/watch?v=pinoLTCdB5w
10 https://www.ajc.com/john-lewis/john-lewis-last-words/GGQ6MKJTIBHGHJ7RQXZVLQFHUA/
11 https://www.sbnation.com/2020/7/31/21349439/nike-ad-all-athletes-created-equal
12 https://www.goodmorningamerica.com/culture/video/tyler-perry-surprises-deserving-cleaning—warriors-georgia-72184742
13 https://youtu.be/7LcLqIHzNkY
14 https://www.nytimes.com/2020/03/24/us/coronavirus-doctor-poetry-boston.html
15 https://www.youtube.com/watch?v=DhS6tuyB7wA&ab_channel=ReelChicagoReel360
16 https://www.nature.com/articles/s41577-022-00725-0
17 https://jewishunpacked.com/yom-kippur-greetings-what-to-say-to-your-jewish-friends-on-yom-kippur/
18 https://www.chabad.org/library/article_cdo/aid/995354/jewish/How-to-Celebrate-Yom-Kippur.htm
19 https://hbr.org/2021/06/5-models-for-the-post-pandemic-workplace
20 https://hbr.org/2022/02/we-need-time-to-rehabilitate-from-the-trauma-of-the-pandemic
21 https://em360tech.com/tech-article/what-happened-to-blockbuster
22 https://www.youtube.com/watch?v=1JR5oEeorbo&ab_channel=TheHellenicAmericanLeadershipCouncil
23 https://aspr.hhs.gov/COVID-19/Therapeutics/Products/Evusheld/Pages/default.aspx
24 https://www.covid19treatmentguidelines.nih.gov/therapies/antivirals-including-

antibody-products/molnupiravir/

https://news.emory.edu/tags/topic/molnupiravir/index.html

25 https://www.covid19treatmentguidelines.nih.gov/therapies/antivirals-including-antibody-products/remdesivir/

https://news.emory.edu/stories/2020/04/coronavirus_emory_helps_lead_research_on_remdesivir/index.html

26 https://www.newsobserver.com/news/local/article259532679.html

27 https://www.holifestival.org/significance-of-holi.html

28 https://timesofindia.indiatimes.com/life-style/events/happy-choti-holi-2022-wishes-messages-quotes-images-facebook-whatsapp-status/articleshow/90274807.cms

29 https://www.hindustantimes.com/lifestyle/festivals/passover-easter-ramadan-2022-fall-simultaneously-101650028357390.html

30 https://wellness.emoryhealthcare.org/our-people-ramadan

31 https://www.nj.com/entertainment/2022/04/passover-and-easter-overlap-in-2022-heres-why-they-have-more-in-common-than-you-might-expect.html

32 https://homegymr.com/micro-tears-in-muscles/

33 https://www.anytimefitness.com/ccc/ask-a-coach/revealed-the-top-reasons-you-may-be-gaining-weight-while-working-out/

34 https://www.blbfilmproductions.com/

35 https://www.usnews.com/news/articles/2015/07/30/desegregation-the-hidden-legacy-of-medicare#:~:text=By%20threatening%20to%20withhold%20federal,hospital%20in%20America%20virtually%20overnight.

36 https://cfmedicine.nlm.nih.gov/physicians/biography_330.html

37 https://www.cnn.com/2019/07/02/business/lee-iacocca-obituary/index.html

38 https://archive.org/details/games_magazine

39 https://tutors.com/lesson/tautology-in-math-definition-examples

40 https://goizueta.emory.edu/faculty/profiles/jeffrey-rummel

41 https://hbr.org/2020/12/podcast-coaching-real-leaders

42 https://murielwilkins.com/about-muriel-wilkins/

43 https://www.youtube.com/watch?v=m2w64Z0p5G8&ab_channel=TPainVEVO

44 https://en.wikipedia.org/wiki/Sully_Sullenberger

45 https://www.investopedia.com/terms/l/law-of-supply-demand.asp

46 https://www.youtube.com/watch?v=w6EblErBJqw&ab_channel=Inc.

47 https://en.wikipedia.org/wiki/Antoine_de_Saint-Exup%C3%A9ry

48 https://www.smartsheet.com/blog/essential-guide-writing-smart-goals

49 https://www.calm.com/app/meditate

50 https://news.emory.edu/stories/2014/07/saintjosephs_sports_cardiologist/campus.html

51 https://news.emory.edu/stories/2019/05/kyle_hammond_named_falcons_head_

Appendix

team_physician/index.html

[52] https://www.heart.org/en/health-topics/heart-attack/about-heart-attacks/heart-attack-or-sudden-cardiac-arrest-how-are-they-different

[53] https://www.sbnation.com/nfl/2023/7/13/23793594/damar-hamlin-bills-training-espy

[54] https://www.npr.org/2023/11/06/1210879092/damar-hamlin-cincinnati-scholarships

[55] https://rohitbhargava.com/

[56] https://www.history.com/this-day-in-history/fosbury-flops-to-an-olympic-record

[57] https://news.emory.edu/stories/2022/10/er_rohit_bhargava_25-10-2022/story.html

[58] https://nonobvious.com/non-obvious-trends/collection/

[59] https://www.youtube.com/watch?v=G4O2Setle1s&feature=youtu.be

[60] https://www.qualtrics.com/experience-management/customer/what-is-voice-of-customer/

[61] https://www.youtube.com/watch?v=wJfZ18KR_GY&ab_channel=EmoryHealthcare

[62] https://www.shelsilverstein.com/

[63] https://www.shelsilverstein.com/9780060256739/a-light-in-the-attic/

[64] https://allpoetry.com/poem/8538827-Reflection-by-Shel-Silverstein

[65] https://news.emory.edu/features/2023/02/er_one_emory_09-02-2023/index.html?utm_source=Emory_Report&utm_medium=email&utm_campaign=Emory_Report_EB_021023

[66] https://news.emory.edu/tags/topic/dalai_lama/index.html

[67] https://www.chia.com/

[68] https://www.cancer.org/cancer/types/breast-cancer/about/how-common-is-breast-cancer.html

[69] https://www.medicalnewstoday.com/articles/322700

[70] https://www.nationalbreastcancer.org/early-detection-of-breast-cancer/

[71] https://www.cancer.org/cancer/latest-news/if-youre-called-back-after-a-mammogram.html

[72] https://www.medicinenet.com/what_percentage_of_abnormal_mammograms_are_cancer/article.htm

[73] https://winshipcancer.emory.edu/about-us/nci-designation.html

[74] https://www.cancer.gov/

[75] https://www.abta.org/tumor_types/glioblastoma-gbm/

[76] https://www.cancer.org/cancer/types/gastrointestinal-stromal-tumor.html

[77] https://winshipcancer.emory.edu/bios/faculty/cardona-kenneth.html

[78] https://www.instagram.com/nicolewalters/?hl=en

[79] https://www.eonline.com/news/1241420/shes-the-boss-nicole-walters-details-how-her-teenage-daughter-beat-cancer#:~:text=%22In%202019%2C%20she%20was%20diagnosed,the%20future%2C%22%20Walters%20revealed.

80   https://www.cbsnews.com/news/mercury-retrograde-2022/

81   https://www.theatlantic.com/science/archive/2022/05/mercury-in-retrograde-astrology-real/643117/

82   https://www.today.com/life/astrology/mercury-retrograde-meaning-rcna14394

83   https://www.thegoodtrade.com/features/what-is-mercury-retrograde/#:~:text=Mercury%20entering%20retrograde%20is%20much,actually%20have%20some%20positive%20effects.

84   https://www.who.int/director-general/speeches/detail/who-director-general-s-opening-remarks-at-the-media-briefing-on-covid-19---11-march-2020

85   https://data.who.int/dashboards/covid19/cases?n=c

86   https://www.hhs.gov/about/news/2023/05/09/fact-sheet-end-of-the-covid-19-public-health-emergency.html#:~:text=Based%20on%20current%20COVID-19,day%20on%20May%2011%2C%202023.

87   https://news.emory.edu/stories/2020/05/coronavirus_emory_icu_outcomes/index.html

88   https://news.emory.edu/stories/2020/11/coronavirus_moderna_vaccine_highly_effective/index.html

89   https://news.emory.edu/tags/topic/molnupiravir/index.html

90   https://dph.georgia.gov/covid-19-status-report

91   https://www.cnn.com/2024/06/28/health/covid-summer-wave/index.html

Acknowledgments

I don't know why but writing my acknowledgments me tripped up. My publisher said not to over think them. But I overthought them.

I looked for good examples in books I own. Nothing inspired me.

I Googled examples. Some felt like a preface, while others were so pithy I got tired thinking of writing something equally as clever. More anxiety set in when I saw one woman's post that she loves reading acknowledgments. "I love to read book acknowledgment pages," said blogger Janet Kobobel Grant, "...the acknowledgments I like best are those in which the author shows that he/she has the mojo to cast a creative eye on this page that often tends toward the unimaginative."

My first few tries felt like a terrible Oscar-winning speech—a never-ending list of names where I'd inevitably leave someone important out by accident.

So, I decided to go back to the stream-of-consciousness approach that worked so well for the Friday emails in this book.

First, I have to thank my mother, Susan Moudy. It was her artful red pen on countless school essays that taught me how to write. I'd get so frustrated by her red markings. So much so I finally wrote an essay like she would. It worked. Much less red pen from my mother and much better grades from my teachers.

My second thanks goes to Cheryl Iverson. I mention her a lot in this book, not only because she is a trusted leader on my team, but this book never would have happened had she not suggested that I send our "Rise to the Call" ad to the team that first week of the pandemic.

And speaking of trusted leaders, I need to thank Sandra Mackey and Carolyn Meltzer for believing in me nearly 20 years ago when they welcomed me to the Emory Healthcare team. As well as my trusted partner in all things legal, Chris Kellner, who has been at my side for 15 years, helping navigate trademark, brand, and intellectual property, including advising on this book.

Then, there's my marketing team at Emory Healthcare. This is a special team. We are a family. Yes, I know all about the work family memes and jokes out there, but it's true. I cannot think of any better way to describe our team.

To my accolade and foreword writers for championing me in this journey, from a childhood family friend to NFL MVP, extended family, mentors, industry colleagues and Emory Healthcare leaders—your support means the world to me.

Much love and gratitude go to my husband Chris and son Josh. They are my rock. Together we weathered the storm of the pandemic, leaning in to our love of the ridiculous, watching cornhole, dodge volleyball and cherry-pit-spitting competitions on ESPN 8 The Ocho when live sports ceased. Though the pandemic stressed us and tried our nerves, we also laughed a lot. Big belly laughs at things both simple and outrageous. Even trying our own hand at cherry-pit-spitting in our front yard. It's a lot harder than it looks, btw.

To my dad, Philip Moudy, who taught me the joy of baseball and introduced me to the incredible world of live in-person sports. He and I also share a wicked love of clever puns and wordplay. And my seesters (nope that is not a typo, but how we've called each other as long as I can remember), Lisa and Kelly. We are sisters, friends, confidantes with too many silly and fun memories to count.

Finally, I want to thank Douwe Bergsma for inviting me into Georgia State University's Chief Marketing Officers Roundtable. It's there I attended a breakfast session where the authors in our group shared their journeys to publishing. I met Jo Ann Herold who nudged me over the edge to contact Jeff Hilimire, founder of Ripples Media. He and Andrew Vogel found my story worth publishing and here we are. My deepest thanks to them and the entire Ripples Media team (Jaye Liptak, Dorothy "DMF" Miller-Farleo and Nicole Wedekind) for their support, dedication and hard work making my dream of being a published author reality.

And, if you've made it this far in my book, my gratitude to you, my readers, for reading it and learning more about a different kind of front-line health care worker, and hopefully a bit about leadership and resilience. Thank you from the bottom of my heart.

About the Author

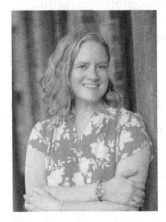

Amy Moudy Comeau, MBA, is an award-winning and acclaimed marketing executive with depth and breadth in health care, non-profit, higher education, and performing arts. As the Vice President of Marketing for Emory Healthcare, she oversees marketing for the most comprehensive academic health care system in Georgia, with decades of experience telling stories and connecting patients, their families, and caregivers with physicians, nurses, and health care professionals.

Throughout her career, which has also included positions at the Lyric Opera of Chicago, The Atlanta Opera, the Rialto Center for the Arts, and Emory University's Nell Hodgson Woodruff School of Nursing, she is known as a collaborative leader adept at building effective cross-functional teams across the enterprise. Her and her team's work has earned in excess of 100 awards for marketing excellence. She is a frequently invited speaker on marketing, leadership and change management.

During her tenure with Emory Healthcare, she led the transition of her team from a marketing communications team to a marketing technology and data-driven team, including growing brand equity to nearly double the company's next closest competitor. She has also incorporated sports partnerships into the organization's broader strategy, leveraging partnerships with the Atlanta Braves (Major League Baseball), Atlanta Falcons (National Football

League), Atlanta Hawks (National Basketball Association), and Atlanta Dream (Women's National Basketball Association).

Amy is a graduate of Northwestern University, with an MBA and Beta Gamma Sigma honors from Goizueta Business School at Emory. She lives in a suburb of Atlanta, with her husband Chris and son Josh. Her weekly writing ritual, which began during the pandemic, continues today.

Other Titles From Ripples Media

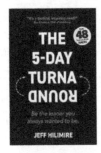
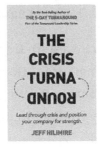
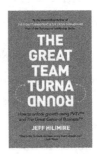

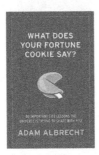
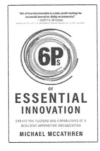
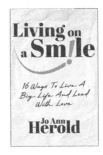

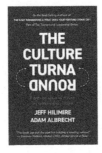
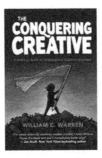
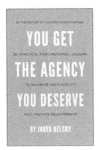

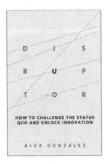
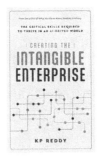

Made in the USA
Monee, IL
25 September 2024